Tuberculosis
AND
AIDS

The Relationship Between Mycobacterium TB and the HIV Type 1

Lawrence L. Scharer, MD

John M. McAdam, MD

With a contribution by Larry Di Fabrizio, MD

SPRINGER PUBLISHING COMPANY

Copyright © 1995 by Springer Publishing Company, Inc.

Springer Publishing Company, Inc.
536 Broadway
New York, NY 10012-3955

Cover design by Tom Yabut
Production Editor: Pamela Lankas

95 96 97 98 99 / 5 4 3 2 1

Library of Congress Cataloging-in-Publication Data

Scharer, Lawrence L.
    Tuberculosis and AIDS : the relationship between mycobacterium Tb and the HIV type 1 / Lawrence L. Scharer, John M. McAdam.
       p.   cm.
    Includes bibliographical references and index.
    ISBN 0-8261-9000-6
    1. Tuberculosis.   2. AIDS (Disease)—Complications.   I. McAdam, John M.   II. Title.
    [DNLM: 1. Tuberculosis—complications.   2. AIDS-Related Opportunistic Infections—complications.   3. HIV-1.   WF 200 S311t 1995]
    RC311.1.S34   1995
    616.9'95—dc20
    DNLM/DLC
    for Library of Congress   95-15168
                                           CIP

Printed in the United States of America

Contents

Acknowledgments

We want to thank Dr. Philip Brickner who encouraged us to write this book. We also want to thank Dr. Ursula Springer and Mr. Matt Fenton of Springer Publishing for their help and patience in producing this book.

Most importantly, we want to thank our wives, Linda and Patricia, for their unconditional support during the 21 months it took us to complete this 6-month project.

L. L. S. and J. M. M.

Contributor

Larry Di Fabrizio, MD, who contributed chapter 3, "Clinical Presentation of Active Tuberculosis," received his medical degree from Washington University School of Medicine in St. Louis in 1984. He completed his medical residency and fellowship in pulmonary medicine in Brigham and Women's Hospital in Boston with a research fellowship in immunology at Columbia-Presbyterian Hospital in New York. Today he is a clinical assistant professor of medicine at New York Medical College, and the director of the pulmonary fellowship training program at St. Vincent's Hospital and Medical Center of New York, where he is also in charge of the pulmonary function laboratory.

Introduction

After a gradual decline for many years in the incidence of active tuberculosis in the United States, there has been a steady increase of new cases since 1985. This has been associated with, and in part is probably secondary to, the coincident epidemic of human immunodeficiency virus (HIV) infection.

It is now well known that infection with HIV causes a reduction in lymphocyte-mediated cellular immunity, allowing infection with tubercle bacilli, both recent and remote, to quickly cause disease. This provides a reservoir of infected and contagious individuals capable of spreading the disease to others in the general community.

Because of the rapid increase in tuberculous rates throughout the United States, especially in the large urban centers, proper diagnosis and effective treatment have become a primary care concern. The days are gone when the few cases of active tuberculosis or the occasional positive tuberculin skin test can be relegated to a specialized pulmonary clinic. Many nurses and physicians trained in the last 10 to 20 years have had inadequate instruction in the diagnosis, management, and control of tuberculosis. Fortunately, there is now much information available on these topics.

The goal of this book is to provide a practical guide for health professionals to help them with the proper diagnosis and treatment of tuberculosis, especially in patients with HIV infection. We will explain the natural history of tuberculosis in normal hosts and then compare this information with what is found when the infection occurs in people with HIV infection. We will review the usual presentation of the disease in both types of hosts, explain how to make a definite diagnosis, discuss available therapy and, finally, discuss public health issues including the management of the noncompliant patient. With the current increase in tuberculosis there has been an additional problem of multidrug-resistant tuberculosis and the spread of these organisms has become a public health emergency, especially in urban environments.

Our discussion is divided into the following topics:

Epidemiology. Chapter 1 examines the distribution and dynamics of disease in populations. We will review the history of tuberculosis from before the discovery of drug treatment up to the present day. The close relationship between tuberculosis and HIV and how this relationship has changed the epidemiology of tuberculosis today will be explored.

Pathogenesis. Chapter 2 reviews the pathologic processes that take place leading to a tuberculous infection and how the infection is usually controlled by cell-mediated immunity. When HIV infection is present it interferes with this defense and promotes the development of active tuberculosis.

Clinical presentations of active disease. The main emphasis of the third chapter is to review the signs and symptoms of "classical" tuberculosis and how they differ in patients with HIV infection. We will review the indications for screening for tuberculosis, explain the difference between infection and disease and how, when disease occurs, it may be primary or reactive in nature. In this section we also discuss pulmonary and extrapulmonary disease and how they are changed when the patient also has HIV infection. Chest x-rays are almost always available in patients suspected of having tuberculosis and are usually abnormal. We will show some examples of what patterns of disease may occur and how they are different when HIV infection is present.

Diagnosis. In order to diagnose infection before the development of disease, we rely on the tuberculin skin test. Chapter 4 reviews the technique, describes how results should be reported, and explains what constitutes a "positive" test in both normal and HIV-infected individuals. Once active disease develops, there is a wide spectrum of tests available. In addition to chest x-rays we will discuss the utility of other tests such as examination of sputum, blood, and other specimens. A tentative diagnosis can be made by finding acid-fast organisms on smears of sputum or other material, but a definite diagnosis is only made by culture of the organism, *Mycobacterium tuberculosis.*

Treatment. Chapter 5 reviews criteria for preventive treatment of those with and without HIV infection. When active disease is present, tuberculous therapy has become more complicated because of increasing numbers of multidrug-resistant (MDR) organisms. Currently available drugs are discussed, combinations suggested, and interpretation of antibiotic sensitivities considered. Special groups such as children, pregnant women, and noncompliant patients who need supervised therapy will also be discussed.

Public health issues. Because of the potential spread of tuberculosis to normal hosts, including health care workers and casual contacts as well as HIV-infected individuals, infection control is discussed in great detail in chapter 6. The management of noncompliant or recalcitrant patients has become an issue of concern all over the United States and we will review various attempts to deal with this problem.

Each year we are seeing more cases of HIV infection and more cases of tuberculosis. We hope this book clarifies this association and provides strategies for recognizing and treating the tuberculosis when it occurs and for preventing its spread. Early diagnosis and appropriate treatment are the keys to the eventual elimination of tuberculosis as a public health hazard.

The Epidemiology of Tuberculosis and Human Immunodeficiency Virus

Epidemiology is the science describing the dynamic relationships between disease and populations. It is concerned with who in a population has a particular disease and why. There are two basic assumptions fundamental to epidemiology. First, human disease does not occur at random. Second, there are causal and preventive factors that can be identified and used to manipulate the spread of disease within a population (Hennekens & Buring, 1987). Epidemiology can be used to discover clues to the etiology of a disease by examining characteristics of those affected. From this examination, the actual etiology of an illness can be discovered. After the etiology of an illness is known, epidemiology can predict who will be most at risk in a community and where to allocate precious resources to best help those at risk. The epidemiology of tuberculosis (TB) led researchers to discover its infectious nature and Dr. Robert Koch to discover *Mycobacterium tuberculosis* as the causative agent in 1882. The clustering of early cases of acquired-immunodeficiency syndrome (AIDS) among gay men, injecting drug users, and blood product recipients led modern researchers to speculate that an infectious agent carried in body fluids was the cause of AIDS. After serologic testing became available in 1985, large surveys showed that AIDS cases were only the tip of the iceberg in a wide spectrum of human immunodeficiency virus (HIV) disease. Finally, the clustering of cases of active tuberculosis among those infected with HIV led scientists to understand the relationship between these two diseases.

TUBERCULOSIS EPIDEMIOLOGY IN THE PAST

Tuberculosis is as old as humanity. Prehistoric remains and Egyptian mummies have shown evidence of tuberculous disease. So many bodies with tuberculous lesions were unearthed in one area of Egypt that it was postulated that there must have been the equivalent of a tuberculosis sanitarium at this site (Dubos & Dubos, 1992). The term *phthisis,* meaning wasting, was coined by the ancient Greeks, although its true etiology was then unknown. The Greeks' precise descriptions still characterize the clinical appearance of active tuberculosis today. The word *tuberculosis,* however, was not seen in print until 1839 (Ayvazian, 1993). It was first used by Schönlein to describe the whole spectrum of tuberculous diseases, previously described as separate entities.

Tuberculosis is a disease of crowding and poverty, and became a public health issue with the rise of modern cities in the 17th century. Writings of the period indicate that 20% of all deaths in England and Wales in 1650 were due to pulmonary phthisis (Dubos & Dubos, 1992). Although tuberculosis had existed earlier, it became a major public health problem when whole families moved to the cities and lived in crowded, tiny, poorly ventilated rooms. These conditions were ideal for the spread of tuberculosis. By the late 19th century, tuberculosis had become a major cause of death in the United States and the rest of the Western world. Some cities in the eastern United States were reported to have tuberculosis death rates of 400 per 100,000 population (Dubos & Dubos, 1992). In the United States, tuberculosis caused more deaths (200 per

100,000 in 1900) than heart disease, cancer, and stroke combined (Noble, 1987). The tuberculosis death rate fell from 200 per 100,000 population in 1900 to 39 per 100,000 in 1945 (see Figure 1.1). It was 1947 before effective antituberculous therapy became available; so this decrease was largely through public health efforts and a general increase in the standard of living. Public health education efforts resulted in early diagnosis and removal of the contagious patient from the household for treatment in a sanitarium.

The writings of the last few centuries reflect the anxiety of the public toward tuberculosis. John Bunyan wrote: "The captain of all these men of death that came against him to take him away was the Consumption, for it was that brought him down to the grave" (Dubos & Dubos, 1991, p. 8). Thomas Young, in a review of what was known about tuberculosis in 1815, wrote: " Of all hectic affections, by far the most important is pulmonary consumption, a disease so frequent as to carry off prematurely about one-fourth part of the inhabitants of Europe, and so fatal as often to deter the practitioner ever from attempting a cure" (Dubos & Dubos, 1992, p. 9).

There were two schools of thought as to the etiology of tuberculosis. Many believed tuberculosis was an inherited disorder, explaining its ability to decimate entire families. In *The Principals and Practice of Medicine,* published a few months before Koch's announcement, Austin Flint and W. H. Welch said that tuberculosis was due to a combination of "hereditary disposition, unfavorable climate, sedentary indoor life, defective ventilation, deficiency of light, and depressing emotions" (quoted in Ayvazian, 1993, p. 4). Others held that tuberculosis was due to a microorganism and therefore spread from person to person. In 1882, Dr. Robert Koch identified the organism known to us as *Mycobacterium tuberculosis* (MTB) as the etiologic agent of tuberculosis. Although the precise mechanism of transmission (inhalation of airborne droplet nuclei) was not known, it was clear the disease could spread from those with active tuberculosis.

A movement began to control tuberculosis. The purpose was twofold. First, to protect the public welfare, it was necessary to remove those persons with active disease from the household. This was done to prevent further spread of infection and disease. Second, once removed from the household environment, those individuals with active disease could receive specialized treatment at tuberculosis sanitaria. These

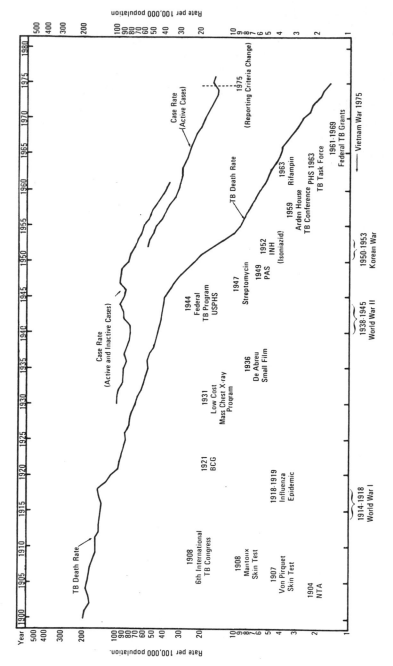

FIGURE 1.1 Tuberculosis, case rates and death rates, United States, since 1900. *Source:* U.S. Department of Health, Education, and Welfare, Public Health Service. (1978). *Extrapulmonary Tuberculosis in the United States.* Centers for Disease Control, Atlanta, Georgia, HEW Publication No. (CDC) 78-8360.

facilities were usually located in the mountains or in rural areas, where it was felt that breathing the pure, rarified air would help combat the disease. In addition, new treatments could be tried to control the disease in the individual. In this pre-antibiotic era, these treatments consisted of therapeutic pneumothoraces, extremely rich diets (up to 12 eggs per day), and plenty of outdoor exposure. The Adirondack style lawn chair was designed for tuberculosis patients to sit outside their cabins. The first electric blanket was used in 1923 to keep tuberculosis patients warm in the outdoor winter air.

The first purpose of sanitaria, to protect the general population from tuberculosis, was an impressive success. The decrease in death rates from tuberculosis in the United States from 1900 to 1946 was not accomplished by anything a doctor could do for an individual patient. The decreased death rate was a result of finding active tuberculosis cases early and removing them from the environment. Removing contagious individuals from households resulted in fewer tuberculous infections, fewer new active cases of tuberculosis and, consequently, fewer deaths. The total number of tuberculosis cases fell rapidly, but until effective antibiotics became available in the early 1950s, individuals with active tuberculosis in 1945 were no more likely to survive than in 1910 (New York City Department of Health, 1982). With the advent of multidrug antituberculous regimens in the early 1950s, tuberculosis became curable, and patients could leave the sanitaria and return to their families with a minimal chance of relapse.

By the 1970s, tuberculosis sanitaria were closed, and treatment was administered in an ambulatory setting. After an initial period of respiratory isolation lasting about 2 weeks, it was found that tuberculosis patients were no longer contagious and no longer represented an infection risk to their household families. But the early promise of ambulatory treatment was jeopardized by noncompliance with long regimens, followed by reactivation of previously treated disease. Patients could only be cured by fairly strict adherence to lengthy regimens of multiple antibiotics with possible side effects. Treatment regimens lasting from 18 to 24 months were not uncommon. In spite of these limitations, the overwhelming majority of patients with tuberculosis were cured. The number of cases of active tuberculosis continued to decline from 137,006 cases in 1948 to 22,201 in 1985. When corrected for the increase in total population during this period the tuberculosis case rate (cases of illness per 100,000 persons at risk) dropped tenfold—from 93.8 to 9.30 per 100,000 (Centers for Disease Control [CDC], 1992d).

EPIDEMIOLOGY OF TUBERCULOUS INFECTION AND DISEASE TODAY

Poverty, Crowd'ng, and Race

Tuberculosis has long been a disease of those living in hardship, forced to share crowded, poorly ventilated homes favoring its spread (Knopf, 1900). It has always been more common in the United States in urban areas than rural ones (CDC, 1991b). Within cities, tuberculosis case rates tend to be highest in areas of the greatest poverty and/or lack of access to medical care. In 1992 in New York City, with an overall tuberculosis case rate of 52 per 100,000 population, the highest cases rates were in the Manhattan Central Harlem (240.2) and the Bronx Mott Haven (168.2) health districts. (New York City Department of Health, Bureau of TB Control, 1993). Individuals belonging to so-called racial or ethnic minority groups—blacks, Hispanics, Asians, and Native Americans—tend to live in these poorer areas, and are usually described as having higher infection and disease rates than whites (CDC, 1992d). It is not clear if this is a result of environmental exposure or if there are immunological differences between various ethnic or racial groups. A study looking at tuberculous infection rate differences between blacks and whites in prisons and nursing homes suggested that blacks have a greater tendency to become infected with *M. tuberculosis* than whites in the same environment (Stead, Senner, Reddick, & Lofgren, 1990). Poverty, however, may contribute to differences in infection and disease rates among minorities. A survey of New York City Board of Education employees in the 1970s showed increasing rates of tuberculin skin test reactivity in zip code areas of New York City corresponding to lower average family incomes (Reichman & O'Day, 1978). The Centers for Disease Control recently issued a figure demonstrating increasing rates of active tuberculosis within zip code areas of the United States corresponding to areas with the lowest household incomes (CDC, 1992a). The poorest members of American society are often members of racial and ethnic minority groups. Their apparently increased rates of tuberculous infection and disease may be more a result of impoverished living conditions than any genetic predisposition, and this remains a controversial topic. The poorest of the poor, persons who are homeless or residents of shelters, single room occupancy hotels, or other marginal living situations have the highest infection and disease rates of any known group based on age, race, sex, or economic status (CDC, 1992c).

Although coinfection with HIV greatly increases the risk of development of active tuberculosis, it is not known if it increases the risk of acquiring a tuberculous infection, although one could probably assume this to be true. To what degree coinfection with HIV and *M. tuberculosis* increases the risk of development of active tuberculosis and the mechanism by which this occurs is discussed later.

Duration and Intensity of Exposure

Tuberculosis goes through two distinct stages in progressing from infection to disease. Infection is transmitted to an individual from an index case of active tuberculosis. The index case is the first case of a contagious disease in a local outbreak. It has been estimated that a hospital worker exposed to an untreated, infectious case of pulmonary tuberculosis would require 600 to 800 hours of exposure to become infected (Riley, 1957). The number of new infections generated by an active case of tuberculosis varies greatly depending on the infectiousness of the source, or index case, the intensity and length of exposure, and also certain environmental factors. It appears that patients with tuberculosis and HIV are no more infectious to household contacts than other tuberculosis patients according to a report from Nunn and colleagues (Nunn et al., 1993). Fortunately, only about 10% of immune-competent hosts with tuberculous infection will develop active disease during their lifetimes. About half of these develop active disease in the first 2 years after acquiring the infection. The remainder develop active disease over the next several years or even decades later. It is only with the development of active disease that others can become infected. There are various medical illnesses that increase the likelihood of progressing to active tuberculosis. These are discussed in chapters 2 and 5.

HIV INFECTION AND TUBERCULOSIS

In 1981, there were reports of unusual pneumonias such as *Pneumocystis carinii* occurring in gay or bisexual men, and sometimes accompanied by a cutaneous malignancy, Kaposi's sarcoma (CDC, 1981). *Pneumocystis carinii* was an organism known to cause pneumonia in patients who were debilitated or immune-compromised because of treatments such as cancer chemotherapy. The men evaluated in these reports had none of the usual causes of immunodeficiency. Kaposi's sarcoma had been known as a slowly growing cutaneous malignancy principally affecting elderly men, who usually died of other causes rather than Kaposi's sarcoma. This condition of impaired immunity became known as the acquired immunodeficiency syndrome (AIDS), and has gone from 189 cases in the United States in 1981 to 339,250 confirmed cases through September 30, 1993. It has caused 204,390 deaths in the United States, and there have been over 2,500,000 cases worldwide since the epidemic began (CDC & World Health Organization, 1993). The etiology of the illness was discovered in 1984 and found to be a retrovirus later named human immunodeficiency virus type 1 (HIV-1, or more commonly, HIV). Presently, while treatable, HIV-1 disease remains a progressive, deteriorating illness, usually resulting in death. Although treatments can delay the onset of severe illness in many, AIDS remains incurable.

In 1983, an association was found between AIDS and tuberculosis. A group of Haitian immigrants in South Florida in whom AIDS developed were more likely to develop tuberculosis than other populations (Pitchenik et al., 1984). It was also noted that cities with the greatest AIDS and HIV disease problems were also among the first areas of the country to show an increase in tuberculosis (CDC, 1986). Still others noted that active tuberculosis seemed to develop as a manifestation of AIDS or HIV infection in those populations traditionally at greater risk for tuberculous infection (Chaisson et al., 1987).

The mechanism by which HIV causes immune deficiency is the selective destruction of CD4 or T-helper cell lymphocytes. These cells normally secrete lymphokines, boosting the ability of macrophages to engulf and destroy mycobacteria and other pathogens (Bender, Davidson, Line, Brown, & Quinn, 1988). Persons with HIV are more likely to progress to active tuberculosis after an initial infection with M. *tuberculosis* than those without an HIV infection (Hopewell, 1993). This arm of the immune system prevents tuberculosis from developing from a primary tuberculous infection in immunocompetent hosts. When cellular (CD4 lymphocyte) immunity is depressed in an individual with a concurrent M. *tuberculosis* infection, the rapid progression to active tuberculosis is much more likely. This was clearly demonstrated by Selwyn and colleagues in a study published in 1989 (Selwyn et al., 1989). They found that during a 2-year period, purified protein derivative (PPD) positive, injecting drug users with HIV infection developed active tuberculosis at the rate of 8% per year. The control group, also injecting drug users, had no cases of active tuberculosis during that period. Keeping in mind the effect of HIV on the individual's immune system, we need to understand what can happen when these results are duplicated on a large scale.

Primary active tuberculosis was thought to have developed in less than 2,500 (13%) of 20,000 persons newly infected with M. *tuberculosis* in 1990. The remainder of the 25,000 cases that year are believed to have been caused by reactivation of dormant or old infections (CDC, 1991a). The presence of many people with compromised cellular immunity increases the number of new tuberculosis cases developing soon after acquiring tuberculous infection. The long latency phase between infection and development of disease is gone, altering the natural history of tuberculosis and resulting in rapid spread. This phenomenon was demonstrated in several well-documented outbreaks which occurred in hospitals (Beck-Sague et al., 1992) and in a supportive residence for those with HIV disease (Daley et al., 1992). Patients became infected and then ill with active tuberculosis within weeks to months rather than the usual years to decades. In one outbreak, patients with severe HIV infection, already on treatment for drug-susceptible tuberculosis, became infected with and developed multidrug-resistant (MDR) tuberculosis. Two recent studies using restriction-fragment-length polymorphism[1] (RFLP) analysis demonstrated

---

[1]RFLP is also known as DNA fingerprinting. Each species of organism shares common base pair sequences of DNA. Within each species there are other areas of the DNA chain that are unique to various strains of the same organism. Two separate cases of tuberculosis that are not the result of transmission of the organism from the first person will have very different RFLP patterns. If a person with active tuberculosis transmits that infection to one or more bystanders and they become ill with active tuberculosis, the RFLP patterns will be a very close or even an exact match.

that one third of new cases of tuberculosis in San Francisco were the result of recent infection, as were 40% of new tuberculosis cases in a section of the Bronx in New York City (Small et al., 1994; Alland et al., 1994). Based on these studies, the treatment of tuberculous infection has taken on a new sense of urgency. A substantial proportion of new cases of tuberculosis may no longer result from the activation of a remote infection. Transmission of tuberculous infection with the rapid emergence of active disease becomes possible when HIV-infected individuals are living in crowded conditions with little or poor access to medical care.

HIV infection is the greatest risk factor for the development of active tuberculosis ever identified. Persons coinfected with HIV and *M. tuberculosis* may be 100 times more likely to develop active tuberculosis than those with simple tuberculous infection (Selwyn et al., 1989). Individuals coinfected with tuberculosis and HIV are 10 times more likely to develop active tuberculosis than persons with any other known form of immune deficiency (Table 1.2, CDC, 1992b). The increased rate of active tuberculosis in those coinfected with HIV-1 and *M. tuberculosis* synergistically leads to further tuberculous infection, and more active tuberculosis.

In the normal propagation cycle for tuberculosis, once a person becomes infected, there is a slight chance of progressing directly to active disease. For every 100 persons infected with *M. tuberculosis,* 10% will eventually develop active tuberculosis. About half of these cases develop within the first 2 years after infection. The risk of developing active disease then decreases sharply, and the remaining 5% will develop active disease over the next several decades (CDC, 1991a). This phenomenon gives clinicians years to discover and preventively treat this latter group.

In those with HIV infection, nearly all who acquire a tuberculous infection may develop active tuberculosis and the active stage will arrive much earlier, on the order of days to weeks or months rather than years or decades (Daley et al., 1992). Both infection and disease can spread more rapidly in such an immune-compromised population. The overall effectiveness of preventive treatment is reduced because there is less time to find and treat those at risk.

On a larger scale, the rise of HIV infection is believed to be at least partly responsible for the failure of plans to eradicate tuberculosis in the United States by early in the next century (CDC, 1989). The dismantling of the public health system on city, state, and federal levels is also a factor in the re-emergence of tuberculosis (Reichman, 1991). Rising national tuberculosis rates over the past several years are illustrated in Figure 1.2. To date, there have been 64,000 more cases of tuberculosis in the United States than would have been expected if prior trends had continued. These were 64,000 extra tuberculosis cases that the already overburdened public health system was forced to absorb.

Throughout the world, the goal of tuberculosis elimination, nearing reality only a few years ago, has now become more elusive. The increase in tuberculosis in the United States noted since 1985 is a small reflection of what has occurred throughout the world. In western Europe, the decreases noted during the 1970s have not been sustained in some countries (CDC, 1993). In eight countries, increasing proportions of new tuberculosis cases are among foreign-born persons from countries with a high prevalence of tuberculosis (CDC, 1993). Among European tuberculosis patients, HIV seroprevalence is generally not known. Case definitions differ between countries, making precise comparisons difficult. The impact of HIV on tuberculosis in Europe may be limited to areas where HIV seroprevalence in tuberculosis is high (e.g., Paris, 12%).

Cases in Africa nearly doubled from 1987 to 1988. Rates of active disease in all Europe, Oceania, Asia, and the Americas increased by 44%, 36%, 26%, and 20%, respectively (Styblo, 1991). Much of this increase is associated with the explosion of HIV disease in these areas. There is a complex interplay of factors responsible for the effects of HIV on tuberculosis in a population (Styblo, 1991; see Table 1.1). Some factors relate to HIV and tuberculosis prevalence in the population. Others

TABLE 1.1 Factors Involved in the Impact of Human Immunodeficiency Virus (HIV) on the Epidemiology of Tuberculosis in a Population

- Prevalence of HIV infection in the community and its trend
- Prevalence of HIV infection in the general population aged 15–49 years
- Breakdown rate from tuberculous infection to active tuberculosis
- Level of and trend in the annual average risk of tuberculous infection
- Detection rate of new and relapse cases of tuberculosis and cure rate of smear-positive cases

Source: Adapted with permission from Styblo, K. (1991). The impact of HIV infection on the global epidemiology of tuberculosis. *Bulletin of the International Union Against Tuberculosis and Lung Disease, 66,* 27–32.

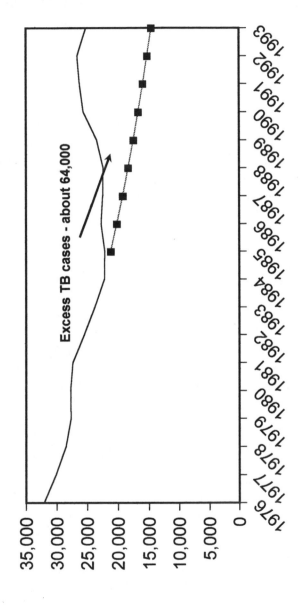

Figure 1.2 Number of reported tuberculosis cases—United States, 1976–1993. *Source:* Centers for Disease Control (1994). Reported Tuberculosis in the United States, 1993. U.S. Department of Services, Atlanta, Georgia.

TABLE 1.2 Risk Factors for the Development of Active Tuberculosis
Among Persons Infected with *Mycobacterium tuberculosis*

Risk factor	Estimated increased risk for tuberculosis compared with persons with no known risk factor (%)
Acquired immunodeficiency syndrome	170.0
Human immunodeficiency virus infection	113.0
Other immunocompromising conditions*	3.6–16.0
Recentness of infection (≤2 years)	15.0
Age of contact (≤5 years and ≥60 years)	2.2–5.0

*For example, diabetes mellitus type 1, renal failure, carcinoma of head or neck, iatrogenic immunosupression.

Source: Centers for Disease Control (1992). Management of persons exposed to multidrug-resistant tuberculosis. *Morbidity and Mortality Weekly Report, 41*, (RR-11), 37–45.

concern the ability of the public health system to detect new active cases of tuberculosis, prevent relapses, and effect cures in a reasonable amount of time.

SUMMARY

Epidemiology first pointed to the infectious nature of tuberculosis and later showed its route of infection. Epidemiologic studies helped establish the infectious nature of HIV-1 and discovered its association with *M. tuberculosis*. We now know that simultaneous infection with HIV and tuberculosis can lead to unprecedented rates of active tuberculosis. Early detection of infection and prompt treatment are more urgent now because of the rapid rate of progression from tuberculous infection to active tuberculosis. Before the emergence of HIV-1 there were often years between the acquisition of infection and the development of active disease, if it developed at all. Now those with dual *Mycobacterium tuberculosis* and HIV-1 infections may progress to active disease in a matter of weeks. Continued epidemiologic surveillance will help guide our prevention, treatment, and control efforts.

REFERENCES

Alland, D., Kalkut, G. E., Moss, A. R., McAdam, R. A., Hahn, J. A., Bosworth, W., Drucker, E., & Bloom, B. R. (1994). Transmission of tuberculosis in New York City. *New England Journal of Medicine, 330,* 1710–1716.

Ayvazian, L. F. (1993). History of tuberculosis. In L. B. Reichman & E. S. Hershfield (Eds.), *Tuberculosis: A comprehensive international approach* (p. 3). New York: Marcel Dekker.

Bender, B. S., Davidson, B. L., Line, R., Brown, C., & Quinn, T. C. (1988). Role of the mononuclear phagocyte system in the immunopathogenesis of human immunodeficiency virus infection and the acquired immunodeficiency syndrome. *Review of Infectious Diseases, 10,* 1142–1154.

Beck-Sague, C., Dooley, S. W., Hutton, M. D., Otten, J., Breeden, A., Crawford, J. T., Pitchenik, A. E., Woodley, C., Cauthen, G., & Jarvis, W. R. (1992). Hospital outbreaks of multidrug-resistant *Mycobacterium tuberculosis* infections: Factors in transmission to staff and HIV-infected patients. *Journal of the American Medical Association, 268,* 1280–1286.

Centers for Disease Control. (1981). *Pneumocystis carinii* pneumonia—Los Angeles. *Morbidity and Mortality Weekly Report, 30,* 250–252.

Centers for Disease Control. (1986). Tuberculosis—United States, 1985—and the possible impact of human lymphotrophic virus type III/lymphadeno-pathy-associated virus infection. *Morbidity and Mortality Weekly Report, 35,* 76–86.

Centers for Disease Control. (1989). A strategic plan for the elimination of tuberculosis in the United States. *Morbidity and Mortality Weekly Report, 38(suppl),* 1–25.

Centers for Disease Control. (1991a). *Core curriculum on tuberculosis.* Atlanta, GA: United States Department of Health and Human Services, United States Public Health Service.

Centers for Disease Control. (1991b). *Tuberculosis statistics in the United States, 1989* (HHS Publication No. CDC 91-8322). Atlanta, GA: United States Public Health Service.

Centers for Disease Control. (1992a). In *HIV-related tuberculosis* (slide presentation). Atlanta, GA: United States Department of Health and Human Services, Division of Tuberculosis Elimination.

Centers for Disease Control. (1992b). Management of those exposed to multidrug-resistant tuberculosis. *Morbidity and Mortality Weekly Report, 41(RR-11),* 37–45.

Centers for Disease Control. (1992c). Prevention and control of tuberculosis among homeless persons. *Morbidity and Mortality Weekly Report, 41*(RR-5), 13–23.

Centers for Disease Control. (1992d). Summary of notifiable diseases 1992. *Morbidity and Mortality Weekly Report, 41*, 60–61.

Centers for Disease Control. (1993). Tuberculosis—western Europe, 1974–1991. *Morbidity and Mortality Weekly Report, 42*, 628–631.

Centers for Disease Control & World Health Organization. (1993). Case watch. *AIDS Clinical Care, 5*(12), 1.

Chaisson, R. E., Schecter, G. F., Theuer, C. P., Rutherford, S. W., Echenberg, D. F., & Hopewell, P. C. (1987). Tuberculosis in patients with the acquired immunodeficiency syndrome: Clinical features, response to therapy, and survival. *American Review of Respiratory Disease, 136*, 570–574.

Daley, C. L., Small, P. M., Schecter, G. F., Schoolnik, G. K., McAdam, R. A., Jacobs, W. R., Jr., & Hopewell, P. C. (1992). An outbreak of tuberculosis with accelerated progression among persons infected with the human immunodeficiency virus. *New England Journal of Medicine, 326*, 231–235.

Dubos, R., & Dubos, J. (1992). *The white plague: Tuberculosis, man, and society* (2nd ed.). New Brunswick, NJ: Rutgers University Press.

Hennekens, C. H., & Buring, J. E. (1987). Definition and background. In S. L. Mayrent (Ed.), *Epidemiology in medicine* (p. 3). Boston: Little, Brown, & Company.

Hopewell, P. C. (1993). Tuberculosis and infection with the human immunodeficiency virus. In L. B. Reichman & E. S. Hershfield (Eds.), *Tuberculosis: A comprehensive international approach* (p. 373). New York: Marcel Dekker.

Knopf, A. S. (1900). The tenements and tuberculosis. *Journal of the American Medical Association, 34*, 1151–1154.

New York City Department of Health. (1982). Tuberculosis 1882–1982, Robert Koch and the discovery of the tuberculosis bacillus. *City Health Information, 22*(1), 1–4.

New York City Department of Health, Bureau of Tuberculosis Control. (1993). *Tuberculosis in New York City 1992, information summary.*

Noble, J. (1987). Tuberculosis and nontubercular diseases. In J. Noble (Ed.), *Textbook of general medicine and primary care* (p. 927). Boston: Little, Brown & Company.

Nunn, P., Mungai, M., Nyamwaya, J., Gicheha, C., Brindle, R. J., Dunn, D. T., Githui, W., Were, J. O., & McAdam, K. P. W. J. (1994). The effect of human immunodeficiency virus type-1 on the infectiousness of tuberculosis. *Tubercle and Lung Disease, 75*, 25–32.

Pitchenik, A. E., Cole, C., Russell, B. W., Fishl, M. A., Spira, T. J., & Snider, D. E., Jr. (1984). Tuberculosis, atypical mycobacteriosis, and the acquired immunodeficiency syndrome among Haitian and non-Haitian patients in South Florida. *Annals of Internal Medicine, 101,* 641–645.

Reichman, L. B. (1991). The "U"-shaped curve of concern. *American Review of Respiratory Disease, 144,* 741–742.

Reichman, L. B., & O'Day, R. (1978). Tuberculous infection in a large urban population. *American Review of Respiratory Disease, 117,* 705–712.

Riley, R. L. (1957). The J. Burns Amberson Lecture: Aerial dissemination of pulmonary tuberculosis. *American Review of Tuberculosis and Pulmonary Diseases, 76,* 931–941.

Selwyn, P. A., Hartel, D., Lewis, V. A., Schoenbaum, E. E., Vermund, S. H., Klein, R. S., Walker, A., & Friedland, G. H. (1989). A prospective study of the risk of tuberculosis among intravenous drug users with immunodeficiency virus infection. *New England Journal of Medicine, 320,* 545–550.

Small, P. M., Shafer, R. W., Hopewell, R. C., Singh, S. P., Murphy, M. J., Desmond, E., Sierra, M. F., & Schoolnik, G. K. (1993). Exogenous reinfection with multidrug-resistant tuberculosis in patients with advanced HIV infection. *New England Journal of Medicine, 328,* 1137–1144.

Small, P. M., Hopewell, P. C., Singh, S. P., Paz, A., Parsonnet, J., Ruston, D. C., Schecter, G. F., Daley, C. L., & Schoolnik, G. K. (1994). The epidemiology of tuberculosis in San Francisco: A population-based study using conventional and molecular methods. *New England Journal of Medicine, 330,* 1703–1709.

Stead, W. W., Senner, J. W., Reddick, W. T., & Lofgren, J. P. (1990). Racial differences in susceptibility to infection by *Mycobacterium tuberculosis. New England Journal of Medicine, 322,* 422–427.

Styblo, K. (1991). The impact of HIV infection on the global epidemiology of tuberculosis. *Bulletin of the International Union Against Lung Diseases, 66,* 27–32.

2

Pathogenesis of Tuberculosis

TRANSMISSION

When people cough or sneeze, airborne droplets also known as droplet nuclei are produced and projected into the air about them. The infectious unit in tuberculosis, *Mycobacterium tuberculosis* (MTB), is carried on these airborne particles. These are small enough (5–10 microns) that they can remain airborne for some period of time and can then be inhaled by a potential host. Larger particles are also produced and may be inhaled but they are usually trapped by the normal defense mechanisms against inhaled particles, the mucociliary blanket, which lines the bronchial tree, and then carried up into the mouth where they are swallowed or expectorated. Infection does not occur in that situation because tubercle bacilli deposited on intact mucosa or skin do not invade tissue.

Transmission of infection is dependent on several factors: (a) the presence of live bacilli in large numbers in the patient's sputum, (b) sputum aerosolization into small airborne particles when the patient coughs, speaks, or even sings (in patients with pulmonary or laryngeal tuberculosis), (c) an appropriate duration of exposure to the infected air, and (d) a susceptible host. Although many people are concerned about a single intense exposure, tuberculosis is not a highly infectious

disease and transmission usually requires close and prolonged exposure to a patient with large numbers of organisms in his/her sputum.
Studies show that casual or limited contact usually does not lead to
infection or disease (Riley, 1967).

PATHOGENESIS

If the tubercle bacilli are inhaled and reach the pulmonary alveoli, a
fairly well-known series of events begins. There are usually only a few
organisms at one site, since larger clumps don't reach the alveolar
space. These organisms are engulfed by the alveolar macrophages normally present and that have this phagocytic function. Some of the
organisms are killed but many remain viable and multiply within the
macrophages and eventually lead to cell death. More cells are now
attracted from the blood stream to the area of infection. These blood-
borne macrophages can ingest the bacilli but usually don't kill them
because they are not activated for this function. Activation requires
lymphocytes, which manufacture lymphokines, as discussed later in
this section.

Granuloma Formation

If activated and stimulated, macrophages can ingest and kill the bacterial organism, but more usually they undergo a morphologic change
into epithelioid cells and begin to aggregate into discrete granulomas.
After some time (1–3 weeks) granulomas are well formed with central
necrosis. As the process progresses, necrotic foci tend to enlarge and
coalesce. There is now necrotic debris surrounded by a layer of epithelioid histiocytes and multinucleated giant cells. This, in turn, is surrounded by zones of mononuclear cells and then by fibroblasts. These
three zones of epithelioid cells, mononuclear cells, and fibroblasts are
called tuberculous granulation tissue.

Granulomas localize the tubercle bacilli within a discrete region of
the lung to prevent further spread of the disease. This lesion may be
grossly visible and the central necrotic material is called *caseation necrosis* because it has a cheese-like appearance. When visible in pathology
specimens or on chest x-rays it is called the *Ghon focus*. It may heal as

the fibroblasts form collagen and scar or the central necrotic material may persist with viable organisms but separated and contained by the fibrous scars. In time it may calcify and if present with a calcified draining lymph node, both seen on chest x-ray, it is called a *Ghon complex*. It is this focus where tuberculosis first started and then healed that can again become active when the patient develops *reactivation tuberculosis*. This can occur many years later or the disease may continue at the time of the primary infection leading to progressive primary tuberculosis.

Macrophage Function

The progress or remission of the disease is determined by the ability of the macrophage to inhibit the growth of the tubercle bacillus. There are variations of response depending on genetic and immunological factors. Hosts vary in ways we do not understand in their ability to fight the tubercle bacillus. As we will discuss throughout this book, coinfection with HIV is the most important and serious problem that can affect the host's response; but long before we knew about HIV infection, other genetic factors were suspected. The possibility exists that even the initial infection may occur more often in certain groups, including those infected with HIV, as well as a greater chance of infection leading to actual disease. The question of race has been raised for many years. Stead, Senner, Reddick, and Lofgren (1990) presented results of their analysis of racial differences in susceptibility to infection by M. *tuberculosis*. They concluded, looking at infection rates among initially tuberculin-negative residents of 165 racially integrated nursing homes in Arkansas, that blacks have about twice the relative risks of whites of becoming infected with M. *tuberculosis*. This was independent of any factors that may affect the progression from infection to active disease.

Lymphocyte Function

The role of the lymphocyte is crucial in the body's defense and, as we will describe later, the impairment of lymphocyte function when infection with HIV occurs can be disastrous. Normally, lymphocytes are attracted from the blood stream to the site of infection by the antigens of the tubercle bacillus. Following exposure to these new antigens to which they now become sensitive, or to other stimulating agents called mitogens, the lymphocytes manufacture and release biologically active substances known as lymphokines. It is these lymphokines that activate and transform the blood-borne macrophages to perform ingestion and killing of tubercle bacilli. Depending on the effectiveness of this process in a given host, the tubercle bacilli may be confined to the lung, spread via the hilar lymph nodes into the bloodstream, or spread directly into the bloodstream by erosion of small blood vessels by the developing tubercles.

Cell-Mediated Immunity and Delayed Hypersensitivity

The process of forming granulomas is called *cell-mediated immunity*, and involves macrophages and T lymphocytes, as opposed to the antibody type of immunity, which involves B lymphocytes. As activated lymphocytes reach a certain concentration, tissue hypersensitivity develops, as expressed by a positive tuberculin skin test. There has been considerable discussion as to whether delayed hypersensitivity and cell-mediated immunity are the same or different endpoints of the tuberculous infection. Dannenburg has been a strong advocate of the view that these two immune host responses are quite different (Dannenburg, 1991). He feels that delayed hypersensitivity works by killing unactivated macrophages in which tubercle bacilli are multiplying. These bacilli are inhibited extracellularly within necrotic sites. Cell-mediated immunity activates macrophages so they can kill and digest bacilli they ingest, an intracellular process. Both of these responses can stop the multiplication of tubercle bacilli. In the first, no growth of tubercle bacilli occurs in dead macrophages, which, as noted earlier, are a major component of solid caseous necrotic debris within the tuberculous granuloma. It is cell-mediated immunity, however, that is more important in controlling the spread of the initial infection and the response that is most affected by intercurrent infection with HIV-1.

Once tubercle bacilli have been inhaled, they usually go to the areas of the lungs that have the greatest ventilation, the middle and lower lobes. Here they begin to multiply and spread to the hilar lymph nodes; there is little tissue reaction until hypersensitivity and cell-mediated immunity develop with activated macrophages forming granuloma. During this initial period there may be spread of tubercle bacilli throughout the body without obvious symptoms, so that it is a silent bacteremia. Depending on the blood supply and oxygen tension in the organs of the body, tubercle bacilli which require oxygen to live and multiply, may or may not cause local disease. The most common site for spread is to the posterior and apical portions of the lung where oxygen tensions are the highest in the body. Other favorite areas for the tubercle bacilli to multiply include brain, kidney, spine, and the metaphyseal ends of long bones.

After 6–8 weeks, cell-mediated immunity is well established. In the areas where the tubercle bacilli have spread, granulomatous inflammation develops to destroy these germs by means of the activated macrophages and/or granuloma form to contain them. As a result, most infected hosts have complete healing of these early tuberculous lesions. If cell-mediated immunity is inadequate to contain the infection, then disseminated disease and/or progressive pulmonary tuberculosis may develop.

Healing via cell-mediated immunity and without the use of chemotherapy is not 100% effective. The primary site of infection in the middle or lower lobes rarely contain viable tubercle bacilli once healing has occurred. The apical foci where the organisms have high oxygen tension is where dormant bacilli can remain viable in adults and then can cause late progression of disease. Adult tuberculosis is usually reactivation tuberculosis, not due to exogenous reinfection. Children, in contrast to adults, are more likely to experience spread from this primary site of infection if the child's immunity is inadequate to halt the disease process.

Adding chemotherapy to the natural immune response significantly reduces the chance of the disease persisting and recurring at a later time. Therapy in tuberculin-positive hosts without apparent disease will be discussed along with other treatments in chapter 5.

Why late progression or recrudescence of foci implanted in the course of the primary infection develops is still unclear, but it is well known to occur in a number of clinical settings, especially with the impaired immunity as we see with HIV infection. Reactivation usually occurs during certain times in the host's life when there is normal lowering of natural resistance, such as adolescence, the postpartum period, and even decades after the primary infection in old age. Other conducive conditions include alcoholism, diabetes, prolonged steroid therapy, malnutrition, cancer, and post-gastrectomy (probably due to associated malnutrition and/or alcoholism) (Table 2.1).

Resistance to New Infection

Usually, previously infected people are resistant to new infection. The previous immunological events cause a quick response to inhaled bacilli. Activated macrophages and lymphocytes quickly respond to contain and eradicate the new infection, assuming that the host's immunity is not impaired. If immunity is impaired, as in the situations noted above, then exogenous infection with a new strain of M. *tuberculosis* can occur. By using a process called *phage typing*, investigators have been able to identify individual strains of *Mycobacterium tuberculosis*. This is done with a bacteriophage or phage that is capable of infecting and lysing different M. *tuberculosis* organisms. This technique can show the presence of one phage type from a source case and its presence in a previously tuberculin-positive host.

A new technique called analysis of restriction-fragment-length polymorphisms (RFLPs) is a method of DNA fingerprinting that has also been used to trace the transmission of particular strains of M. *tuberculosis* during various outbreaks of tuberculosis in hospital or shelter settings (Small et al., 1993). The RFLP technique provides evidence of

TABLE 2.1 Medical Conditions that Increase the Risk of Development of Clinical Tuberculosis Once Tuberculous Infection Has Occurred

- HIV infection
- Silicosis
- Abnormal chest radiograph showing fibrotic lesions
- Diabetes mellitus
- Prolonged corticosteroid therapy
- Immunosuppressive therapy
- Hematologic and reticuloendothelial diseases
- End-stage renal disease
- Intestinal bypass
- Post-gastrectomy
- Chronic malabsorption syndromes
- Carcinoma of the oropharynx and upper gastrointestinal tract
- Bodyweight 10% or more below ideal

Source: Centers for Disease Control/American Thoracic Society (1991, April). *The Core Curriculum on Tuberculosis* (2nd ed.).

spread of infection from a known source case to other patients under treatment for another strain of *M. tuberculosis*. In general, however, it is still more likely that a previous infection reactivates than that a new infection occurs. Unfortunately, the more immunosuppressed the patient, the more likely the possibility of acquiring new infections.

Bacille Calmette-Guérin (BCG) Vaccination

The use of bacille Calmette-Guérin (BCG) vaccination, introduced over 70 years ago, is based on the assumption that infection of the host with a nonpathogenic tuberculous organism will stimulate the immunologic process described earlier. Bacille Calmette-Guérin is a live attenuated vaccine derived from a culture of a virulent strain of *Mycobacterium bovis*, which loses its virulence through serial subculturing but will cause tuberculin hypersensitivity to develop. The host should then have activated macrophages and lymphocytes ready to battle the *Mycobacterium tuberculosis* organism if inhaled following exposure to a source case. Its effectiveness, however, has been the subject of considerable debate because protection from the vaccination has varied widely in different trials, in part due to variation in the vaccine used. It is not currently used in the United States, where the emphasis has been on repeated tuberculin skin testing and treatment of tuberculin conversion with chemotherapy, but it is used widely in other countries either in infancy or following the start of school. Recently, a meta-analysis of the published literature (Colditz et al., 1994) demonstrated that BCG reduces the risk of tuberculosis by 50% on the average. The CDC has recommended its use only for tuberculin-negative infants and children who have continued exposure to multidrug-resistant tuberculosis or who simply cannot take isoniazid and suffer ongoing tuberculous exposure. Institutional outbreaks, especially with the emergence of multidrug-resistant tuberculosis, have raised the question of broadening the use of BCG in the United States. The use of the vaccine, however, still has not gained much acceptance in the United States, where most experts in the field still use tuberculin skin test reactions to guide therapy. This attitude may change in the future if multidrug-resistant tuberculosis is not controlled. For BCG to be effective, it has been assumed but never proven that the recipient should develop a positive tuberculin skin test that usually lasts a decade or longer.

The administration of BCG vaccine to HIV-infected persons is contraindicated because of its potential to cause disseminated disease.

A positive tuberculin skin test that is the result of infection with M. *tuberculosis* usually lasts longer, but will also disappear with time. It is assumed that the positive test is due to the presence of live organisms in the host (Rodkey, 1965), without any evidence of disease or repeated exposure to new infections. There is a slow (about 5% per year) loss of tuberculin reactivity in normal hosts in an affluent society with a low prevalence of tuberculosis and little chance for re-exposure. It has been demonstrated that a newly infected host who takes chemotherapy may lose tuberculin reactivity; probably other healthy nonreactors completely overcome the infection so that they lose specific tuberculin hypersensitivity. These people are then presumably at risk to develop newly acquired exogenous infection.

A small proportion of people skin tested will not initially react to the test material but will react a few weeks later if tested again, due to a booster effect which recalls T-cell memory. A positive skin test that requires this booster effect presumably has the same significance as a test which is positive the first time. This is discussed further in chapter 4, which covers diagnostic procedures.

PROGRESSION TO CLINICAL DISEASE

Pulmonary Tuberculosis

More than 90% of the time, individuals are asymptomatic at the time of their primary infection. Most will develop a positive tuberculin skin test as evidence of their newly developed delayed hypersensitivity and have normal chest x-rays and no evidence of disease on physical examination. Occasionally the x-ray will show focal calcifications and/or calcified primary lower lobe lesions. If present with hilar lymph nodes these are known as a Ghon complex.

Years ago, almost all cases of primary tuberculosis occurred in children but we now see it in all age groups. There are four broad syndromes described in symptomatic patients: (a) pneumonia with fever, nonproductive cough, and patchy infiltrates on chest x-rays, (b) pleurisy with effusion, (c) direct progression to upper lobe disease, and

(d) extrapulmonary tuberculosis as a result of progression of the primary infection.

Postprimary, also called reactivation tuberculosis, is more common and is the most frequently seen clinical form as will be described in the following chapter.

Extrapulmonary Tuberculosis

About 20% of cases in the United States initially present in extrapulmonary foci in immunocompetent hosts. Except in children, there may be a long latency period between the first episode of infection and the extrapulmonary presentation. These syndromes are discussed in great detail in chapter 3 on clinical presentations.

HIV AND IMMUNODEFICIENCY

Since the virus causing acquired immunodeficiency syndrome (AIDS) was first recognized in the early 1980s, it has been called various names but is now uniformly known as the human immunodeficiency virus (HIV-1). The presence of this infection leads over time to AIDS. The hallmark of this syndrome is the loss of T lymphocytes with the CD4+ surface marker caused by invasion and destruction by HIV-1.

There are two major groups of lymphocytes. They are T cells (thymus dependent lymphocytes or T lymphocytes) and B cells (bone marrow derived lymphocytes or B lymphocytes). These B cells are involved with the production of antibodies, an important part of our immune system, but one which probably does not play much part in the body's normal response to tuberculosis. The T cell, however, is the primary player in the development of cell-mediated immunity, which controls, among other things, infection with *M. tuberculosis*. During their maturation, T cells develop surface markers including CD4+. (CD stands for cluster of differentiation.) T cells with this marker are also called "helper cells." Those with the CD8+ are known as suppressor or killer cells.

The loss of T-cell function reduces lymphokine production which in turn compromises macrophage function. As discussed earlier, it is the activated macrophage, stimulated by the T cell, which is the body's normal response to tuberculous infection. The activated macrophage is able to engulf and kill mycobacteria, but it needs the stimulation of lymphocytes to perform this task.

Human immunodeficiency virus (HIV-1) is part of a family of retroviruses in which genetic material is stored in ribonucleic acid (RNA) rather than deoxyribonucleic acid (DNA). Once HIV-1 enters a cell, the RNA is copied by a preformed reverse transcriptase contained within the virus. The consequences of the integration of HIV-1 proviral DNA into the host's own DNA are crucial: The infected cell, as long as it lives, will always harbor the virus in a latent state. Initially, when the virus was discovered, it appeared that only 1 in 1,000 CD4+ cells were infected because the virus could slip into the cell showing no signs of outside activity. The effect on the immune system was well known, however, and probably due to the fact that the virus actually inhabits 20% to 30% of CD4+ cells. Thus, there is a quantitative as well as a qualitative loss of T-cell function. The CD4+ lymphocyte is the primary target for HIV infection because of the virus' affinity for the CD4+ marker. These cells coordinate a number of important immunologic functions and the loss of these functions results in the progressive impairment of the immune response. The multiple clinical manifestations of the disease we call AIDS results primarily from the infectious and neoplastic complications of the loss of the normal immune response. There is a strong association between the development of life-threatening opportunistic illnesses and the absolute number or percentage of CD4+ lymphocytes.

Throughout the world, pulmonary tuberculosis is the most common type of tuberculosis in people with HIV infection. When tuberculosis occurs early in the course of HIV infection, the clinical picture is usually no different than in the normal host. Seventy-five to one hundred percent of tuberculosis is pulmonary when the disease develops before other opportunistic infections. It does signal immunologic impairment, however, and the presence of tuberculosis in any organ, pulmonary or extrapulmonary, in someone with HIV infection meets the current CDC definition of AIDS. Although there may be no other markers of HIV infection, the disease spreads more quickly (Daley et al., 1992) than in normal hosts. Infected patients with pulmonary tuberculosis have CD4+ counts ranging from 250–500 cells/mm^3. In comparison, studies of HIV-infected people with extrapulmonary TB usually have CD4+ counts below 250 and often below 100.

Reactivation of Latent Tuberculosis

Most cases of tuberculosis which have been seen in patients infected with HIV have been presumed to be reactivation of latent tuberculosis because these cases occurred among members of groups with a high incidence of underlying tuberculous infection, for example, Haitians and intravenous drug users (IVDU). In 1989, Selwyn et al. presented data showing that in HIV-infected persons, tuberculosis most often results from the reactivation of tuberculous infection and that the use of isoniazid chemoprophylaxis blocked the development of active disease. These patients were previously infected, had dormant infection which became active when their immunity was unable to control the infection. If they took prophylactic drug therapy, the organisms were killed and disease did not occur.

On the other hand, Braun et al. showed spread of newly acquired tuberculous infection in a prison inmate population who were also HIV-infected (Braun et al., 1989). The development of active tuberculosis in previously uninfected HIV-infected patients can also occur following exposure to a contagious source case. As we will discuss later, the clinical presentation is different with a picture of primary, disseminated tuberculosis. It has been suggested that HIV-infected individuals are more likely to acquire tuberculous infection when exposed to *M. tuberculosis* (Daley et al., 1992) but this is still unproven.

Most work in this field has focused on the relationship of the clinical manifestations of tuberculosis to the level of CD4+ cell counts in patients with HIV infection. For example, Jones et al. in 1993 evaluated clinical and laboratory features of 97 HIV-infected patients with tuberculosis (Jones et al., 1993). They concluded that markers of severe cases of tuberculosis, such as extrapulmonary tuberculosis, including positive blood cultures for *M. tuberculosis,* occurred in 70% of their patients when the CD4+ count fell below 100 mm^3. Features dependent on delayed-type hypersensitivity such as positive tuberculin skin tests and tuberculous pleuritis were more common in patients with higher CD4 cell counts.

In subsequent chapters we will discuss clinical presentation, diagnosis, and treatment in the HIV-infected population.

REFERENCES

Braun, M. M., Truman, B. I., Maguire, B., DiFerdinando, G. T., Wormser, G., Broaddus, R., & Morse, D. L. (1989). Increasing incidence of tuberculosis in a prison inmate population: Association with HIV infection. *Journal of the American Medical Association, 261,* 393–397.

Colditz, G. A., Brewer, T. F., Berkey, C. S., Wilson, M. E., Burdick, E., Fineberg, H. V., & Mosteller, F. (1994). Efficacy of BCG vaccine in the prevention of tuberculosis. Meta-analysis of the published literature. *Journal of the American Medical Association, 271,* 698–702.

Daley, C. L., Small, P. M., Schecter, G. F., Schoolnik, G. K., McAdam, R. A., Jacobs, W. R., Jr., & Hopewell, P. C. (1992). An outbreak of tuberculosis with accelerated progression among persons infected with the human immunodeficiency virus. *New England Journal of Medicine, 326,* 231–235.

Dannenburg, A. M. (1991). Delayed type hypersensitivity and cell-mediated immunity in the pathogenesis of tuberculosis. *Immunology Today, 12,* 288.

Jones, B. E., Young, S. M. M., Antoniskis, D., Davidson, P. T., Kramer, F., & Barnes, P. F. (1993). Relationship of the manifestations of tuberculosis to CD4 cell counts in patients with human immunodeficiency virus infection. *American Review of Respiratory Disease, 148,* 1292–1297.

Riley, R. L. (1967). The hazard is relative. *American Review of Respiratory Disease, 96,* 623–625.

Rodkey, G. W. (1965). Chemoprophylaxis in certain positive tuberculin reactors with special reference to reversion to negative and the clinical and public health aspects thereof. *American Review of Respiratory Diseases, 92,* 316.

Selwyn, P. A., Hartel, D., Lewis, V. A., Schoenbaum, E. E., Vermund, S. H., Klein, R. S., Walker, A., & Friedland, G. H. (1989). A prospective study of the risk of tuberculosis among intravenous drug users with immunodeficiency virus infection. *New England Journal of Medicine, 320,* 545–550.

Small, P. M., Shafer, R. W., Hopewell, P. C., Singh, S. P., Murphy, M. J., Desmond, E., Sierra, M. F., & Schoolnik, G. K. (1993). Exogenous reinfection with multidrug-resistant *Mycobacterium tuberculosis* in patients with advanced HIV infection. *New England Journal of Medicine, 328,* 1137–1144.

Stead, W. W., Senner, J. W., Reddick, W. T., & Lofgren, J. P. (1990). Racial differences in susceptibility to infection by *Mycobacterium tuberculosis*. *New England Journal of Medicine, 322,* 422–427.

3

Clinical Presentation of Active Tuberculosis

Larry Di Fabrizio, MD

Few disorders may affect so many organs, mimic so many diseases, and have confounded so many clinicians as disease caused by *Mycobacterium tuberculosis*. This organism has been known to afflict both animal and man since antiquity. Its manifestations were recognized as early as 4000 BC and its clinical features were first documented in Sanskrit medical records (Keers, 1978). However, it was not until 1882, when Koch identified this organism, that direct clinical-pathologic correlation could be made.

Early on in the human immunodeficiency virus (HIV) epidemic, it was recognized that the impairment of immune function induced by HIV infection predisposes individuals to a variety of infections. The HIV infection also altered the clinical presentation and course of these infections, and in many instances, complicated their therapy. Infection with *M. tuberculosis* illustrates each of these points. Namely, patients with HIV infection have increased susceptibility to tuberculosis. It may occur early in the course of HIV infection, and is frequently the initial manifestation of AIDS. However, there may be difficulty in diagnosis due to increased frequency of atypical presentations. Lastly, it has also been shown that there has been an increased frequency of drug-resistant tuberculosis among HIV-infected individuals, with devastating results.

The development of drug-resistant strains of tuberculosis has further increased the urgency for early clinical recognition, isolation, and initiation of appropriate therapy. This chapter attempts to describe both the common and uncommon clinical syndromes that M. *tuberculosis* may cause in both the immunocompetent and HIV-infected host.

CLINICAL SYNDROMES

The clinical manifestations of tuberculosis (TB) depend upon the mechanism of infection, the extent and anatomical location of the disease, the presence of co-morbid diseases, and the immune status of the host. Tuberculosis has also been clinically categorized as recent infection (or primary) and reactivation (or postprimary), as well as pulmonary and extrapulmonary.

Primary Tuberculosis

In the vast majority of cases, as reviewed earlier, tuberculosis is transmitted by inhalation of droplet nuclei to the lower two thirds of the lung. Over the ensuing several weeks after an initial inoculation, the bacilli are phagocytosed. They may also travel to regional lymph nodes via lymphatics, or distant sites via hematogenous spread. Cell-mediated immunity induces an inflammatory reaction which contains and destroys the tuberculi and local tissue. These phenomena are similar in the child, the neonate, and the adult; however, clinically important differences should be recognized.

Children

Tuberculosis was among the leading causes of death in children in the early 1900s. Fortunately, this grim situation has not been the case for several decades. In the United States, patients under 20 years old comprised only 7.6% of all cases of tuberculosis in 1987. However, approximately 40% of these cases were children less than 5 years old. As in adults, immune status and socioeconomic factors are important risk factors in assessing risk of exposure and development of active disease. Infants and young children may be at increased risk of infection because of a relatively immature immune system and intense intimate contact with the primary infecting case. Children are usually infected by an adult or adolescent in the immediate household. This may include a parent, grandparent, sibling, or some other individual who commonly shares the caretaking responsibilities of the child. Socio-economic risk factors are more striking in children than adults since nearly 80% of childhood tuberculosis patients are members of racial and ethnic minorities. The incidence of tuberculosis in nonwhite children is five times greater than among white children. Blacks, Hispanics, American Indians, and Alaskan Natives comprise the majority of cases. Not surprisingly, densely populated urban areas are also associated with higher attack rates of tuberculosis. Certain geographical areas also appear to serve as pockets of tuberculosis for children. In particular, the states of California, Texas, New York, New Jersey, and South Carolina comprised almost half of all cases reported in 1987 (Abernathy, 1987). The most severe problem has occurred in the city of New York, where the incidence of childhood tuberculosis increased 97% from 1989 to 1990. Virtually the entire increase has occurred in children age 4 years old and younger, with black and Hispanic children comprising the majority of the cases (New York City Department of Health, 1991).

In infants and children 3 years or younger, the tissue reaction and clinical course differ from most adults. The tubercle bacilli quickly multiply in the air spaces and are carried to the regional lymphatics and pulmonary veins where they are subsequently distributed to the systemic circulation. The hematogenous spread of tuberculi to brain, bones, kidney, mesenteric lymph nodes and abdominal organs is also more common than in adults. The increased incidence of meningeal and miliary disease in primary TB in childhood must be recognized.

Most children manifest nonspecific symptoms of fever, cough, weight loss, and failure to thrive. Physical exam is also nonspecific. Fever and tachypnea are the most common findings. The examination of the chest is frequently unrevealing. However, on occasion there may be focal wheezes or decreased breath sounds in areas of bronchial obstruction and atelectasis. The rest of the physical exam may be normal or notable for adenopathy and hepatosplenomegaly. The history of exposure and the presence of a positive skin test for tuberculosis are among the most helpful clinical findings.

The chest x-ray is also a useful tool. Regional lymph node involvement, with hilar and paratracheal adenopathy is a common manifestation of primary pulmonary tuberculosis in childhood. Caseation necrosis and resorption followed by rapid calcification of the primary lesion (Ghon lesion) and regional lymph node (Radke complex) are common radiographic patterns seen in children, yet seldom seen in adults. In contrast, primary tuberculosis may also become progressive and cause lobar consolidation, multifocal spread from intrabronchial contamination, or bronchial obstruction with atelectasis from caseous debris or lymphatic compression. Rarely, severe pneumonitis may lead to extensive parenchymal destruction with cavity formation and bronchiectasis, even with appropriate therapy. In older children, as in adults, the infection frequently passes unnoticed. Occasionally, it produces pleurisy with effusion, cervical lymphadenitis, miliary tuberculosis, or meningitis (Turcios & Evans, 1989).

Tuberculosis in HIV-infected children has been recognized in urban areas where both tuberculosis and HIV infection are current problems. In a study of nine children, ages ranging from 6 months to 7 years (median age, 3.5 years), prolonged fever, cough, and anorexia were the most common complaints, and only one patient had a positive tuberculin test (Khouri, Mastrucci, Hutto, Mitchell, & Scott, 1992). Four of the nine patients had evidence of extrapulmonary tuberculosis and the median survival after the diagnosis of tuberculosis was only 20 months. These findings support the need for a high index of suspicion for tuberculosis in HIV-infected children with prolonged fever and respiratory complaints.

Neonates

An unfortunate by-product of the urban tuberculosis crisis is an increased frequency of congenital and neonatal primary tuberculosis infection. As expected, the mechanism of infection is most commonly by inhalation of droplet nuclei. However, ingestion or aspiration of infected membranes or amniotic fluid, and hematogenous spread from the umbilical cord have also been documented.

The clinical presentation of tuberculosis in the newborn is similar to that caused by bacterial sepsis and other congenital infections. Symptoms may be present at birth, but typically develop by the second or third week of life. The most common manifestations include respiratory distress or dyspnea, fever, poor feeding and weight gain, lethargy and irritability, and failure to thrive. Physical exam often demonstrates fever, tachypnea, and tachycardia. Lymphadenopathy, hepatosplenomegaly and abdominal distention are frequently noted. Occasionally, ear discharge or skin lesions are noted. The lung exam is commonly normal or demonstrates focal rales consistent with bronchopneumonia. The purified protein derivative (PPD) skin test is invariably negative, although it may become positive after 1 to 3 months. The chest x-ray is frequently abnormal and demonstrates a miliary pattern in half of the cases. As in the child, adenopathy and parenchymal infiltrates are commonly present.

The clinical course is marked by poor response to antibacterial antibiotics. On many occasions, the only clue to diagnosis is the presence of known or suspected tuberculosis or pulmonary symptoms in the mother or contacts. The diagnosis may be confirmed by smear or culture results obtained from gastric washings, tracheal and middle ear secretions, and spinal fluid. Occasionally, biopsy of bone marrow, liver, or lung are required to establish the diagnosis. Unfortunately, the rare complication of tuberculosis in pregnancy frequently goes unrecognized, and is associated with high infant mortality.

Pregnancy

The interaction between pregnancy and tuberculosis has been debated for many centuries. In fact, Hippocrates first suggested that pregnancy had a beneficial effect on tuberculosis. The hormonal changes associated with pregnancy, and an enlarging uterus, which may induce collapse of pulmonary cavities in the lower lobes, were speculated to deter the development of tuberculosis during the mid-19th century. In contrast, during the 20th century through the prechemotherapy era, several uncontrolled studies suggested an adverse effect of pregnancy on tuberculosis progression. It subsequently became clear that the anatomic extent of disease, the radiographic pattern, and the susceptibility of the individual patient were the main determinants of outcome with tuberculosis, rather than the pregnancy itself (Vallejo & Starke, 1992).

Tuberculosis in women of childbearing age has been on the rise in large urban centers. In New York City the incidence of TB has been reported to be as high as 19 to 39 per 100,000, with the majority of cases occurring among blacks and Hispanics. If unrecognized and not appropriately treated, tuberculosis is associated with miscarriage, prematurity, and increased infant mortality. However, with adequate therapy, the prognosis of the pregnancy should not be adversely affected (Good, Iseman, Davidson, Lakshminarayan, & Sahn, 1981).

The clinical manifestations of tuberculosis in pregnancy is similar to the nonpregnant individual (to be discussed in detail below), and is directly related to the extent and anatomic location of the disease. As expected, cough, weight loss, fatigue, and fever are the most common symptoms. Hemoptysis, a dramatic presentation of pulmonary tuberculosis, occurs in less than 20% of patients, while 20% of patients may have no significant complaints. Extrapulmonary involvement of tuberculosis is uncommon and occurs at the same rate as the general population, approximately 5% to 10% of cases. The PPD skin test is usually positive, unless there is a concomitant immune defect (e.g., HIV infection). Diagnosis is frequently established on clinical grounds and confirmed by culture of sputum in the majority of cases.

The Adult

In the normal adult host, primary tuberculosis may be asymptomatic and go unrecognized. In some instances, a mild illness with fever and malaise may develop. A nonproductive cough may be the only respiratory symptom. In most instances, the initial phase of tuberculosis infection goes undetected. The primary site of infection heals by a combination of resolution, fibrosis, and calcification (Dannenberg, 1993).

Due to the occult nature of primary tuberculosis in adults, a chest x-ray is not commonly obtained. However, when performed, a primary lesion may be seen in any bronchopulmonary segment. Most commonly, the abnormalities lie in the middle or lower lung, which are the areas of greatest ventilation. Regional or hilar adenopathy may be found, but with lower frequency than in primary tuberculosis of childhood. Interestingly, this common finding in children is more frequently noted in the young black adult. As stated previously, the primary foci and regional lymph node (Ghon and Radke complexes) heal and have a tendency to calcify. Rarely, normal adults develop massive hilar and mediastinal adenopathy or compression of major bronchi leading to obstructive atelectasis or focal consolidation.

In approximately 5% of all infected individuals, control of the replicating organism is inadequate, and disease occurs within 1 year of infection. The ability of the host to respond to the organism is greatly reduced by coexisting diseases such as diabetes mellitus, hematologic or reticuloendothelial malignancy, or silicosis. Infection with HIV-1 and immunosuppressive drugs, such as corticosteroids, cytotoxic drugs, and cyclosporine, which suppress cell-mediated immunity, greatly increase the risk of disease progression. In these instances, the defenses are overwhelmed and the patient may develop an overt clinical infection, which may include a localized pneumonitis, pleural effusion, progressive adenopathy, and dissemination of disease. As a rule, the active primary lesion in the adult is difficult to distinguish from a lesion of reactivation tuberculosis, and can be documented only by observation of recent or concomitant tuberculin conversion.

Primary Tuberculosis in HIV-Infected Individuals

The HIV-infected individual with primary pulmonary tuberculosis is more likely to come to clinical recognition. However, unlike the normal host, atypical presentations with extensive pulmonary and extrapulmonary organ involvement is the rule. These patients may have constitutional symptoms of prolonged fatigue, fever, anorexia, and weight loss. Respiratory symptoms of persistent nonproductive cough and, later, exertional dyspnea are commonly seen. Chest pain in association with pleuritis is occasionally noted, but hemoptysis is less commonly seen than in non-HIV patients.

The physical examination may be notable for other stigmata of HIV infection, namely, oral thrush, wasting, and adenopathy. Clubbing, a common finding in chronic suppurative infections, is not usually present in the HIV-infected patient. The examination of the chest may be normal or show rales and egophony, signs of alveolar consolidation. There may be decreased breath sounds and pleural rubs associated with moderate-sized pleural effusions. The abdominal exam may show hepatosplenomegaly, as is the case in patients with miliary tuberculosis.

As in the child, the chest x-ray may demonstrate significant hilar and mediastinal adenopathy. The lung parenchyma may reveal infiltrates in any bronchopulmonary segment, although the mid-lung fields are more common in primary infection. Upper lobe distribution, which is the rule in reactivation tuberculosis, is uncommon in primary tuberculosis. Similarly, cavitation is less common in HIV-infected individuals. Dense alveolar infiltrates mimicking bacterial pneumonias are fairly common. Primary pulmonary tuberculous infection, as in reactivation tuberculosis, may progress to miliary involvement of the lung, with small nodular infiltrates. However, the frequency of this is considerably greater in the HIV-infected patient.

Reactivation (Postprimary) Tuberculosis

Once the immune response has controlled the proliferation of the tubercle bacilli, the tuberculous lesions regress and heal. The organisms enter a latent phase where they may persist in small numbers as intracellular pathogens. Unless the persisting organisms begin to rapidly multiply and cause a reactivation of infection, the patient can remain asymptomatic for life.

The risk of developing reactivation tuberculosis infection varies considerably from person to person. A detailed history and clinical exam is indicated to stratify risk of reactivation. Patients with prior exposure to tuberculosis and current HIV infection are at highest risk of reactivation with a frequency of up to 10% per year developing clinically active disease. Among high-risk patients for reactivation are non–HIV-infected individuals with indirect evidence of a large inoculum exposure. This includes individuals with radiographic changes consistent with prior tuberculosis exposure, and close contacts of patients with active tuberculosis. In addition, patients with impaired immunity other than HIV infection are also at higher risk of reactivation. Alcoholics, diabetics, victims of silicosis, postgastrectomy patients, patients with end-stage renal disease, patients receiving immunosuppressive drugs, patients with malignancy, especially lymphoproliferative disorders, are all immunosuppressed to varying degrees, and should be given special consideration for tuberculosis reactivation. Finally, PPD-positive adolescents and young adults represent patients at increased risk of reactivation of tuberculosis due to long lifetime possibility of reinfection.

Because clinical tuberculosis may develop from either direct pro-gression of the initial infection or recrudescence of a dormant lesion, it is frequently difficult to make this clinical distinction. Classically, the most striking clinical features of reactivation tuberculosis are the absence of recent exposure, known prior exposure, the tendency toward clinical chronicity, and cavitation and fibrosis of pulmonary parenchyma. However, many of these classical findings are not com-monly observed in HIV-infected patients. Fortunately, there is no dif-ference with regard to choice of initial therapy based on the mode of infection. Therapeutic choices are based on likelihood of drug resis-tance, which will be addressed elsewhere.

Clinical Spectrum of Pulmonary Tuberculosis

General Clinical Features

The clinical manifestations of pulmonary tuberculosis are highly vari-able. As expected, they depend on the intensity and extent of involve-ment, as well as the host's ability to contain and eradicate its spread. Signs and symptoms are due to both systemic effects of infection and localized involvement. The lung, as portal of entry for the bacillus, is by far the most commonly affected organ.

Mode of Presentation

The pattern of onset may take many different forms. An insidious onset with nonspecific constitutional symptoms, which are frequently fol-lowed by the development of respiratory complaints, is the most com-mon presentation. Some patients develop a catarrhal syndrome with cough, sputum, and coryza-like symptoms of rhinorrhea and nasal congestion. The presentation of a flu-like syndrome or acute febrile ill-ness is not uncommon in debilitated individuals, especially HIV-infected patients. Occasionally, isolated dramatic symptoms such as hemoptysis, severe pleuritic chest pain, or hoarseness may distress and frighten patients into seeking medical attention.

History

Constitutional Symptoms. Constitutional symptoms are common and are frequently the earliest indicator of infection. Fever, sweats, malaise, and weakness are invariably present to some extent. In some instances abdominal symptoms may dominate, associated with anorexia, indigestion, amenorrhea, and rapid weight loss. Fever, which may go unnoticed by the patient, may be high, but is usually less than 40 °C. Sweating may be profuse and characteristically occurs at night. Neuropsychiatric symptoms such as emotional lability, irritability, depression, and headache are common but generally not severe.

Respiratory Symptoms.   Cough is the most common symptom of pulmonary tuberculosis. It is usually nonproductive at first, but as sloughing of caseous lesions occurs, the patient develops mucopurulent sputum. The quantity and character of the sputum is variable, however, it is generally yellow in color and neither foul-smelling nor thick. In severe cases with extensive bronchial inflammation, or cavity formation with tracheobronchial communication, the sputum may be copious and highly infectious in nature. Bronchorrhea with foul smelling, purulent sputum is not commonly observed unless there has been the development of bronchiectasis with superimposed bacterial infection. Bronchiectasis secondary to tuberculosis is usually confined to the upper lobes, making mucus impaction and secondary bacterial infection less likely. In fact, the majority of cases of TB-associated bronchiectasis are "dry," that is, not associated with sputum production.

Expectoration of blood, or hemoptysis, a common symptom of pulmonary tuberculosis does not necessarily indicate active infection. When associated with acute infection it commonly appears as blood-streaked sputum. However, larger volumes of hemoptysis may be seen in multiple settings: (a) bronchiectasis secondary to healed tuberculosis, (b) rupture of an artery in the wall of an old cavity (Rasmussen's aneurysm), (c) erosion of blood vessels in an old cavity due to secondary aspergillosis, atypical mycobacterial or bacterial infection, and (d) erosion of a calcified lesion or broncholith into an airway. In most cases, this bleeding averages 1 to 2 ounces and is self-limited. On rare occasion, however, the bleeding may be massive and associated with shock, asphyxia, and fatality.

Chest pain is seen in a variety of syndromes associated with tuberculosis. Most commonly, sharp or dull pain on inspiration, or pleurisy, is present in patients with pneumonitis and adjacent pleural inflammation. The pain is localized to the innervation of the intercostal nerve adjacent to the inflamed parietal pleura. However, an inflammatory process involving the central portion of the diaphragm will be referred to the ipsilateral shoulder. Severe sharp pleuritic chest pain in association with dyspnea may indicate a spontaneous pneumothorax. Radicular pain across the chest may be associated with spinal tuberculosis. Rarely, precordial pain has been described in patients with pericardial tuberculosis. More common are chronic chest pain syndromes with intermittent dull chest pain, ache, or tightness which are generally nonexertional. These pains are thought to be the sequelae of chronic pleural inflammation and scarring.

Shortness of breath, or dyspnea, is commonly seen during the febrile illness and may be severe in patients with respiratory insufficiency. Yet, in the chronic or dormant stages of infection, dyspnea is uncommon in the absence of extensive parenchymal destruction, large pleural effusions, endobronchial obstruction, or pneumothorax.

Hoarseness and associated neck pain are uncommon symptoms in patients with pulmonary tuberculosis. However, when present, they suggest involvement of the larynx, a highly contagious form of tuberculosis.

Physical Examination

The physical examination, although nonspecific for tuberculosis, is required to assess the severity and extent of infection. Fever in association with tachypnea and tachycardia is commonly seen.

Examination of the chest may be normal or only demonstrate posttussive rales in areas of apical fibrosis. Localized wheeze, rhonchi, and altered breath sounds may reflect endobronchial involvement, which may not have radiographic correlation. Increased fremitus, bronchial breath sounds, egophony, and rales may signify areas of consolidation or atelectasis due to bronchial obstruction. Dullness to percussion and decreased breath sounds are found in effusions, which are commonly of moderate size. Amphoric breath sounds may be heard over cavities. In patients with longstanding pulmonary disease or prior thoracoplasty, there may be noticeable asymmetry in the appearance and excursion of the chest wall, muscular atrophy, and tracheal deviation.

The remainder of the physical exam should demonstrate the presence of past or currently active extrapulmonary tuberculosis. The skin may reveal hyperpigmentation in the setting of hypotension, suggesting adrenal insufficiency. Erythema nodosum may be seen in primary tuberculosis, but usually only in children. Clubbing is rare, but may be seen in patients with a chronic clinical course. The examination of the eyes may demonstrate conjunctivitis, and rarely iritis and chorioretinitis. Assessment of the reticuloendothelial system may demonstrate adenopathy and hepatosplenomegaly. Examination of abdomen and genitourinary systems may reveal a rectal fistula, or the presence of uterine or prostatic and epididymal infection, in females and males, respectively. Skeletal tuberculosis may be manifested by tenderness over the back and spine. Neurological examination revealing an abnormal mental status, cranial palsies and nuchal rigidity may signify tuberculous meningitis.

Laboratory Studies

A variety of hematological manifestations have been described. Mild leukocytosis and anemia are the most common. In patients with pulmonary tuberculosis, leukocytosis to $12,000–15,000/mm^3$ is seen with an increase in polymorphonuclear leukocytes and early band forms. Monocytosis and eosinophilia may also be seen. Elevation of the erythrocyte sedimentation rate, acute phase reactants, and hypergammaglobulinemia are common but nonspecific findings. In rare instances, leukemoid reactions have been noted, but when there is disseminated disease and bone marrow involvement, leukopenia and pancytopenia may develop.

Lymphopenia and anergy may be seen and are common manifestations of HIV infection. Importantly, reactivation of pulmonary tuberculosis in HIV-infected patients commonly occurs with CD4 T-cell counts of $200–500/mm^3$. In contrast, other AIDS-defining conditions, such as *Pneumocystis carinii* pneumonia and *Mycobacterium avium-intracellulare,* are typically noted when CD4 T-cell counts are less than $200/mm^3$, and less than $50/mm^3$, respectively.

Catabolism and weight loss, which are also common manifestations of HIV infection, are the most common metabolic aberrations in tuberculosis. Low total cholesterol and albumin are frequently noted. Alkaline phosphatase and elevated gamma glutaryl transferase may be seen with liver involvement. However, the most common metabolic effect of tuberculosis, aside from weight loss, is hyponatremia. It is commonly associated with the syndrome of inappropriate antidiuretic hormone (SIADH). This complication had been associated with a poor prognosis, possibly due to the fact that SIADH is associated with extensive lung and central nervous system involvement. In addition, patients with adrenal insufficiency may present with hyponatremia, hyperkalemia, and a metabolic acidosis. These patients are frequently volume depleted and have an appropriate increase in antidiuretic hormone (ADH).

Arterial blood gases generally show well-maintained oxygenation. However, when progressive infection or acute miliary tuberculosis occurs in HIV-infected patients, significant hypoxemia may be found.

Pulmonary function testing in patients with tuberculosis is nonspecific. Patients with chronic tuberculosis, as manifested by parenchymal destruction or pleural fibrosis, frequently develop a restrictive ventilatory defect with decreased lung volumes and a proportional decrease in diffusing capacity. In patients with extensive chronic pulmonary tuberculosis, severe derangements of gas exchange and pulmonary hypertension may develop, and lead to cor pulmonale.

Chest Radiography

The chest x-ray, although not diagnostic for pulmonary tuberculosis, is unlike other laboratory data in that it may provide strong presumptive evidence of past or current tuberculosis infection. It is necessary in assessing the location, extent and, frequently, the pathogenesis of tuberculosis infection. Chest x-rays may also be a guide to the stability of the underlying disease. The terms "old" or "fibrotic" should be avoided when interpreting a single x-ray because they may often be misleading. However, a chest x-ray that is unchanged over a 3- to 4-month interval generally indicates "old" tuberculosis or another disease. The presence of any persistent infiltrate in an elderly individual must include tuberculosis among the diagnostic possibilities.

In patients with clinical findings suspicious for tuberculosis a standard posterior-anterior and lateral radiograph should be obtained. Specialized views may also be obtained to aid in diagnosis, as clinically indicated. For example, the apical-lordotic or oblique views may allow visualization of infiltrates which are obscured by bony structures. Tomography, which was commonly used to delineate the nature of parenchymal nodules, cavities, and calcifications, has been replaced by computed tomography (CT). Computed tomography scanning is especially helpful in assessing adenopathy in the hilum and mediastinum.

Furthermore, high-resolution CT scanning is useful in the definition of bronchial stenosis, broncholiths, and bronchiectasis, and has supplanted the use of bronchography. Magnetic resonance imaging (MRI) is rarely indicated in the work-up of tuberculosis. However, magnetic resonance imaging is superior to computed tomography in assessing involvement of the spine, the central nervous system, the vascular structures, as well as the very apex and base of the lung.

The Non–HIV-infected Patient.   Non–HIV-infected patients with reactivation of tuberculosis may show foci of recrudescence at sites of primary infection (the Ghon complex) or sites of early hematogenous seeding (the lung apex). The most common radiographic pattern is the development of a soft 1–2 cm infiltrate at the apical or subapical and posterior portions of the upper lobes. There is a slow progression at first with development of nodular densities as caseous necrosis and tubercle formation develops. As intrabronchial spread of infection occurs, there is radiographic progression of infiltrates. Healing and fibrosis may occur in some areas as extension occurs in others. This leads to the development of pulmonary fibrosis and volume loss or atelectasis of lung parenchyma. As extensive caseous necrosis and sloughing of parenchyma occurs cavitation may develop. If the patient is severely immunosupressed, there may be large areas of lobular or lobar consolidation, which subsequently may undergo necrosis and cause large cavities. If disease progression is slow, there is a greater tendency for fibrosis of the pulmonary parenchyma. This scarring leads to extensive volume loss, thickening of the pleural space, and distortion of the relationship with mediastinal structures. Ultimately, parenchymal and lymphatic calcification, retraction of the hilus, deviation of the trachea and vascular structures are late sequelae.

   Thus far we have been discussing the initial discovery of tuberculosis on a chest x-ray. Often, however, we see patients many years after the diagnosis and treatment have been completed. Their chest x-rays may be normal, but usually show extensive scarring or destruction. Finally, results of surgical procedures as discussed under therapy may be present.

The HIV-Infected Patient.   The radiographic appearance of tuberculosis in HIV-infected individuals is directly related to the degree of immunosuppression (Yamaguchi & Reichman, 1992). Patients who are HIV-infected yet have relatively intact immune function present with findings characteristic of reactivation tuberculosis, such as upper lobe infiltrates and cavitation. Less often, x-rays reveal lower lobe infiltrates, mediastinal adenopathy, and pleural effusions. In a small prospective study of tuberculosis in 13 HIV-infected patients, with a median CD4 count of 324/mm^3, the radiographic findings demonstrated focal infiltrates in 6 (46%), cavitary lesions in 4 (31%), diffuse infiltrates in 6 (46%), and a miliary pattern in 1 (8%; Theuer et al., 1990). In this study, there was no significant difference in the radiographic presentation when compared to non–HIV-infected patients. In contrast, among the HIV-infected patients that are anergic, have low CD4 counts, and had prior opportunistic infections, the radiographic manifestations of tuberculosis are commonly atypical.

In patients with advanced HIV-induced immunosuppression, chest radiographic findings are frequently similar to those seen in primary tuberculosis. Infiltrates may be focal or diffuse. There may be nodular densities. Occasionally, the nodules may coalesce and develop into large infiltrates, which may mimic a bacterial pneumonic process. Intrathoracic adenopathy is also common in tuberculosis in advanced HIV infection. Disseminated disease with pleural effusions and miliary patterns are frequently seen. Cavitation, however, is rare. This is possibly due to the lack of inflammatory process combined with the ineffective remodeling and repair typical with advanced immunodeficiency. In one study the chest radiographs of HIV-infected patients were suggestive of mycobacterial disease in 85% of patients (Modilevsky, Sattler, & Barnes, 1989). Hilar adenopathy (42%), pleural effusion (29%) and predominantly upper lobe infiltrates (25%) were the most common abnormalities noted. However, a miliary pattern (13%) and cavitation (6%) were uncommon. Rarely, tuberculosis may mimic *Pneumocystis carinii* pneumonia. In some instances the x-ray is normal, as may be the case in endobronchial tuberculosis. Therefore, a high index of suspicion for tuberculosis is always necessary in a febrile HIV-infected patient.

Differential Diagnosis. The chest x-ray, although not diagnostic of tuberculosis, is most helpful in the development of a differential diagnosis in the febrile HIV-infected patient (Murray & Mills, 1990). Hilar adenopathy and pleural effusions are common findings in tuberculosis, Kaposi's sarcoma, and non-Hodgkin's lymphoma. They are rare in cytomegalovirus and *Pneumocystis carinii* infection. Bilateral upper lobe infiltrates and thin-walled cavities, which may mimic tuberculosis, have been reported in patients with *P. carinii* pneumonia who were receiving aerosol pentamidine for prophylaxis. Focal air space consolidation, which is fairly common in tuberculosis, is more frequently seen in bacterial pneumonia, Kaposi's sarcoma, and fungal disease such as cryptococcosis. A diffuse fine reticulonodular or miliary pattern is the most common presentation of *P. carinii*. Coccidioidomycosis and histoplasmosis are fungi that commonly mimic tuberculosis. However, presentation with diffuse infiltrates is more typical, extrapulmonary manifestations are prominent, and epidemiology and serology frequently aid in the diagnosis of these entities. In contrast to adults, children with diffuse infiltrates commonly represent involvement with lymphocytic interstitial pneumonitis. Finally, cavitation may be seen in patients with necrotizing bacterial pneumonia, nocardia, and fungi (especially aspergillus), as well as tuberculosis. Although uncommon in advanced HIV-infected patients with tuberculosis, cavitation is generally associated with positive acid-fast smears and is readily diagnosed.

Some examples of changes we have discussed are presented in Figures 3.1 through 3.8.

Tuberculin Skin Test

The tuberculin skin test, which is discussed in detail in chapter 4, has been the traditional method for demonstrating infection with *Mycobacterium tuberculosis*. In HIV-infected individuals, the response to tuberculin is dependent on the degree of immunosuppression. Anergy, the absence of a reaction despite prior exposure, commonly occurs when CD4 T-cell counts are less than 200 cells/mm^3. Therefore, an understanding of the patient's immune function and prior probability of infection must be integrated into the assessment of tuberculin skin testing.

Diagnosis

The history, physical exam, skin testing, and chest x-ray may raise the clinical suspicion for tuberculosis. The diagnosis is established, however,

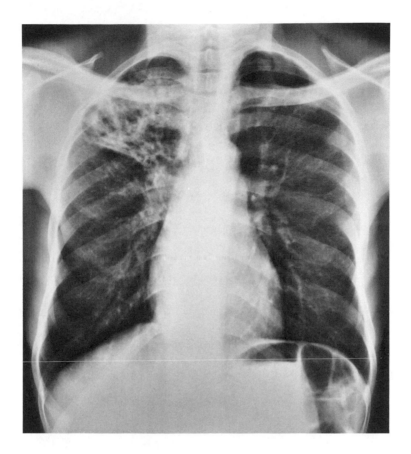

FIGURE 3.1   Reactivation tuberculosis in the right upper lobe with cavity formation (HIV-negative patient).

by isolation of M. *tuberculosis* on culture (details discussed in chapter 4). Specimens for examination for acid-fast bacilli and mycobacterial culture include sputum, bronchoalveolar lavage, transbronchial biopsy, needle aspiration, or biopsy of bone marrow, lymph node, or other involved sites. Culture of blood, urine, cerebrospinal fluid, stool, pleural, and other body fluids may be helpful in selected cases (American Thoracic Society, 1990).

Analysis of sputum with acid-fast smears and culture is the standard method of confirming the diagnosis of pulmonary tuberculosis, as

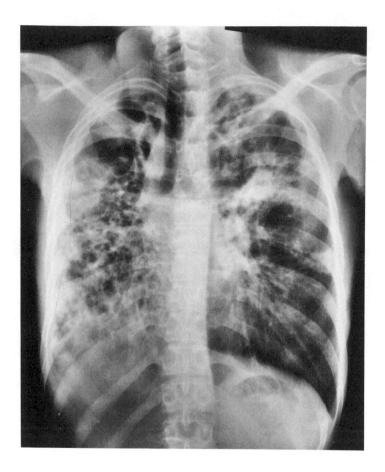

FIGURE 3.2   **Extensive scarring in both lungs with bullae formation following therapy for tuberculosis (HIV-negative patient).**

discussed in chapter 4. Sputum smears are positive in 50%–80% of those with active pulmonary tuberculosis. In severely immunocompromised HIV-infected patients the yield of sputum smears may be significantly decreased. When patients with HIV infection who presented with findings typical of reactivation tuberculosis were compared to non–HIV-infected patients, there was no significant difference in the frequency of positive smears (47% vs. 51%, respectively; Theuer et al., 1990).

The difficulty in identification of tuberculosis in HIV-infected patients may lead to important delays in diagnosis. Late recognition of tubercu-

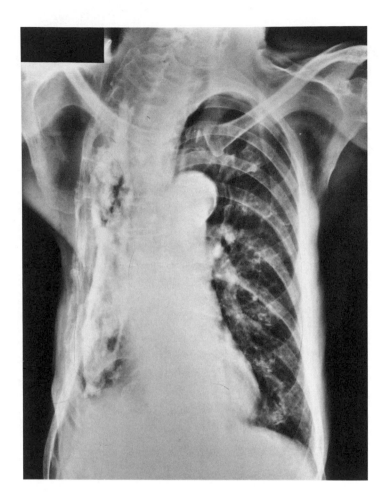

FIGURE 3.3 Total collapse (thoracoplasty) of the right chest done in the prechemotherapy era with subsequent calcification of the pleura.

losis has been shown to be associated with increased morbidity and mortality, and in some instances, nosocomial spread of infection (Kramer, Modilevsy, Waliant, Leedom, & Barnes, 1990). Therefore, patients with clinical and radiographic findings suggestive of tuberculosis should be placed in respiratory isolation, have a minimum of three sputum samples analyzed for acid-fast bacilli, and empiric institution of antituberculosis therapy.

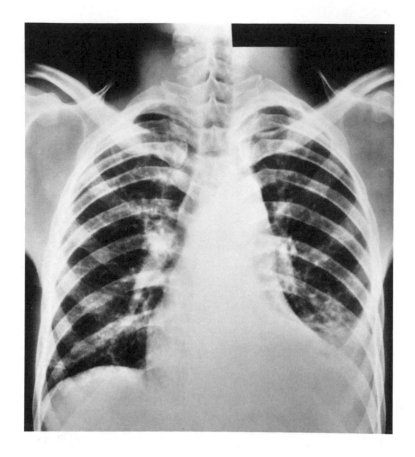

FIGURE 3.4   Tuberculous pleural effusion in the left chest (HIV-positive patient).

Clinical Spectrum of
Extrapulmonary Tuberculosis

The clinical manifestations of extrapulmonary tuberculosis are highly diverse and may reflect involvement of virtually every organ. Often clinically occult, extrapulmonary tuberculosis requires an astute search for diagnostic clues to avoid delays in diagnosis, increased morbidity, and possible disease transmission. Despite the innumerable clinical findings, there are several distinct and recognizable syndromes. Involvement of the central nervous system, pleura, lymphatics, geni-

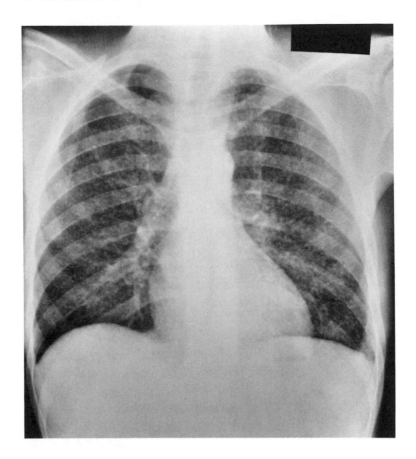

FIGURE 3.5 **Diffuse miliary tuberculosis (HIV-positive patient).**

tourinary tract, and bones, as well as miliary disease, are among the most common syndromes of extrapulmonary tuberculosis.

Like pulmonary tuberculosis, the importance of extrapulmonary disease has changed considerably over the course of this century. In the 1900s, miliary tuberculosis was a disease of infancy and childhood. As public health measures improved, it became a disease of the elderly, although in the medically underserved, childhood cases continued to be observed. Prior to the HIV epidemic, the number of cases of extrapulmonary tuberculosis in the United States remained at approximately 4,000 per year. In 1984, prior to the effect of the HIV epidemic, the

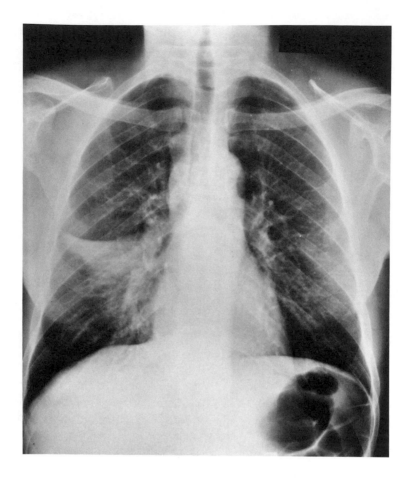

FIGURE 3.6   Right middle lobe infiltrate due to active tuberculosis (HIV-positive patient).

number of tuberculosis cases were steadily declining. The lung was the exclusive organ of involvement in 83.8% of cases, and 16.2% where extrapulmonary, while only 4.2% of cases had combined pulmonary and extrapulmonary involvement. Surprisingly, from 1984 to 1989, the number of cases of extrapulmonary tuberculosis increased by 20%, as compared to a 3% increase in the total number of tuberculosis cases. This dramatic increase in extrapulmonary tuberculosis has been attributed to the high frequency of extrapulmonary tuberculosis in HIV-infected patients (Braun et al., 1990). Specifically, extrapulmonary disease

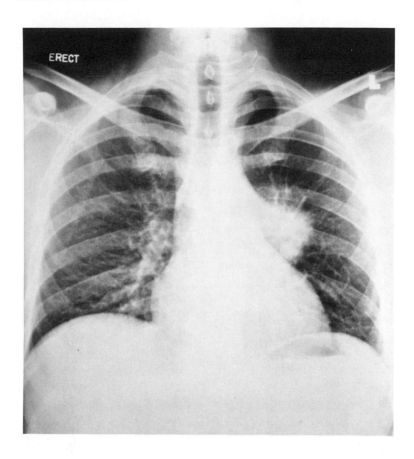

FIGURE 3.7   Left hilar lymph node enlargement with small left pleural effusion, both due to active tuberculosis (HIV-positive patient).

occurs in more than 70% of patients with TB and pre-existing AIDS or AIDS diagnosed soon after the diagnosis of tuberculosis, but in only 24% to 45% of patients with tuberculosis and early HIV infection. Thus, extrapulmonary tuberculosis appears to be more common in patients with more severe HIV-induced immunosuppression (Shafer, Kim, Weiss, & Quale, 1991).

Miliary Tuberculosis

Miliary tuberculosis is the prototype of extrapulmonary TB, since it is caused by the hematogenous dissemination of the tubercle bacilli,

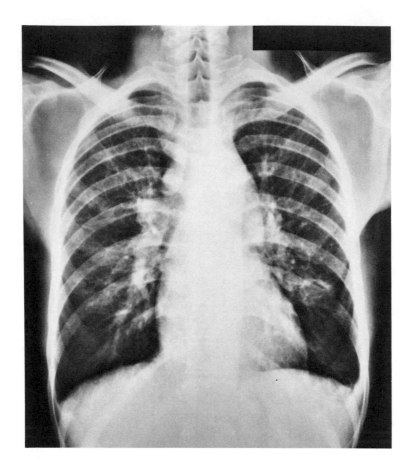

FIGURE 3.8   Patchy bilateral infiltrates, right hilar enlargement, and a small left pleural effusion, all due to tuberculosis (HIV-positive patient).

either at the onset of the initial infection or at the time of endogenous reactivation, resulting in the invasion of various sites. As stated earlier, the state of host resistance determines the nature, extent, and severity of dissemination. Any condition that adversely affects cell-mediated immunity can predispose to extrapulmonary tuberculosis, including starvation, immunosuppressive drugs, organ failure, lymphoproliferative disorders or advanced solid tumors, and certain viral infections, most notably HIV.

The clinical presentation of miliary TB may be acute, subacute, or chronic. In the acute form there is a large and continued infusion of mycobacterial organisms in the bloodstream. The patients appear to be very sick with high fevers, chills, severe weakness, and rapid weight loss. Cough is not prominent but dyspnea occurs as the patient develops progressive pulmonary involvement. Commonly, a bacterial infection is suspected. Routine blood cultures, however, are negative and there is no response to an initial course of antibacterial therapy. In the subacute form of miliary tuberculosis, smaller numbers of bacilli escape into the bloodstream on an intermittent basis. Clinically, there is more prolonged fever and fatigue, slow weight loss, and extrapulmonary organ involvement. Chronic miliary tuberculosis results from sporadic seeding of blood, and may result in isolated organ involvement. This form of miliary tuberculosis may be the most difficult to identify and may remain undiagnosed for months to years (Munt, 1971).

As expected, patients with severe immunosuppression are most likely to present with an acute clinical presentation. A subacute or chronic presentation, on the other hand, is more likely in elderly patients with reactivation tuberculosis, due to a slow decline in immune function.

Constitutional complaints of fever, weakness, malaise, anorexia, wasting, and weight loss are the most common findings when histories are taken. Initially, dyspnea with exertion may be the only respiratory complaint. Cough is not prominent, but when present is usually nonproductive. However, progressive dyspnea and rapid progression to pulmonary insufficiency may occur if tuberculosis goes untreated. In some instances, however, infection may present in an indolent fashion or with fever of unknown origin. Occasionally, patients present with headache and mental status changes or localizing symptoms of direct organ involvement, for example, bone pain.

The physical exam commonly demonstrates fever, tachypnea, wasting, hepatomegaly, adenopathy, and splenomegaly. The chest exam may be normal or reveal diffuse inspiratory rales, when there is extensive pulmonary involvement. On occasion, there may be signs of serositis with pleural and pericardial effusions, or ascites. Rarely, the finding of a choroidal tubercle, a granuloma located in the choroid of the retina, may be the clue to diagnosis of disseminated tuberculosis. This lesion can be gray, gray-white, or yellow with irregular margins, and is usually one fourth or less of the diameter of the disk. It is generally found within 2 optic disk diameters of the nerve head, but may be found more peripherally.

As expected, the laboratory findings are nonspecific. Characteristically, tuberculosis involves the bone marrow and may be associated with a mild decrease in the white blood count and anemia of chronic disease. However, findings ranging from a leukemoid reaction to aplastic anemia have been reported. In rare instances, disseminated intravascular coagulation may be found. Biochemical evaluation occasionally reveals hyponatremia secondary to SIADH or adrenal insufficiency. In the absence of adrenal or extensive pulmonary disease, hyponatremia may suggest pituitary or hypothalamic involvement. Liver chemistries frequently show an "infiltrative" pattern with a modest increase in alkaline phosphatase, gamma-glutaryl transferase, and serum glutamic oxaloacetic transaminase (SGOT; now known as asparate aminotransferase [AST]) with a mild increase in bilirubin. The PPD skin test is negative in 25% to 50% of patients. In severely immunocompromised and HIV-infected individuals, anergy is the rule rather than the exception.

The chest x-ray remains a valuable tool in the diagnosis of miliary tuberculosis. In patients with reactivation tuberculosis that subsequently disseminates, the characteristic apical infiltrates or cavities may be a clue of prior tuberculosis infection. However, in some patients, the initial chest radiographs may be normal. As the infection progresses, hematogenous spread of tuberculosis induces a diffuse fine nodular, interstitial abnormality. The term *miliary* is applied to this appearance because the nodules are about the size of millet seeds (approximately 2 mm in diameter). In patients with HIV infection or children with disseminated tuberculosis, adenopathy is also a common concomitant finding. As noted earlier, pleural or pericardial effusions are occasionally also present.

The radiographic interstitial abnormality is associated with several physiologic derangements. There is a slow decrease in lung compliance, which leads to diminished lung volumes and a restrictive ventilatory defect, a decreased diffusing capacity, and hypoxemia on pulmonary function testing. In patients with rapidly progressive or untreated miliary tuberculosis, the loss of pulmonary compliance is associated with an increased labor of breathing, progressive tachypnea, hypoxemia, and respiratory failure (Heffner, Strange, & Sahn, 1988).

The diagnosis is established by identification of acid-fast bacilli or isolation of *M. tuberculosis* from any number of available sites. Autopsy series have shown that the liver, lungs, adrenals, and spleen are the

Lymphatic Tuberculosis

Lymphatic tuberculosis, a less common manifestation of tuberculosis in immunocompetent adult patients, has become a common mode of presentation in HIV-infected individuals. Prior to the HIV epidemic, lymphatic tuberculosis comprised 27.5% of extrapulmonary cases, and less than 5% of the total cases of tuberculosis. In contrast, adenopathy is noted in approximately two thirds of patients with AIDS and tuberculosis. Tuberculous adenopathy is observed in one half of cases of combined pulmonary and extrapulmonary tuberculosis in AIDS, and is even more common in isolated extrapulmonary tuberculosis, occurring in up to 80% of cases.

There are clear clinical distinctions between HIV- and non–HIV-related tuberculous lymphadenopathy. As noted earlier, intrathoracic adenopathy is more common among normal children with primary tuberculosis. However, among adults, females, particularly Asian and Pacific Islanders, are more likely to develop adenopathy. The nodes affected are overwhelmingly anterior or posterior cervical, and supraclavicular. In up to 80% of cases, only the superficial nodes of the neck are involved. However, lymph nodes anywhere may be affected, and need not be contiguous.

Mycobacterial infection of cervical lymph nodes is known as scrofula. This disease has become uncommon in the United States since the elimination of tuberculous cattle and the pasteurization of milk. It is not only seen with *M. tuberculosis;* in some cases it is due to *M. scrofulaceum, M. kansasii,* or *M. avium-intracellulare,*[1] therefore requiring culture and speciation to make a definitive diagnosis.

---

[1]A small but increasing proportion of pulmonary and extrapulmonary mycobacterial infections are caused by organisms other than *M. tuberculosis*. They are usually referred to as "atypical" but are best classified as "nontuberculous" mycobacteria (NTM). They were first identified soon after Robert Koch's discovery of the tubercle bacillus in the last century but it wasn't until the 1950s that they were classified based on laboratory culture characteristics. Although acid-fast on stained smears, with current culture techniques as described elsewhere, including DNA probes, they are easily separated from *M. tuberculosis.*

The most important of this group in patients with HIV infection is the *Mycobacterium avium* complex, which can cause disseminated disease in immunocompromised hosts. In normal hosts the most common type of involvement is pulmonary infection. It is beyond the scope of this book to list all known members of this group, the usual patterns of disease they cause, and appropriate treatment. Most important is to remember that they are not believed to be spread by human-to-human transmission and are therefore not contagious. Furthermore, isolation from sputum may not mean disease but only colonization of the respiratory tract. When found in usually sterile locations, they are more significant.

Typically, the non–HIV-infected patient presents with painless swelling of one or more lymph node groups. Systemic complaints are uncommon unless there is evidence for tuberculosis at another site. As the infection progresses the groups may become inflamed, matted, and occasionally rupture. Lymph node rupture may lead to a sinus tract, which may be difficult to heal. In children with tuberculous adenitis one may observe massive intrathoracic adenopathy which may compress bronchi and lead to atelectasis, infection, or bronchiectasis. Very rarely has upper airway obstruction been observed in patients with cervical tuberculosis. Tuberculous adenitis may obstruct lymph flow and lead to the development of pleural effusions and ascites. These effusions are typically protein-rich exudates. Occasionally, they are chylous, and consist of milky white fluid which has a high triglyceride content.

In contrast, patients with HIV and tuberculous adenitis commonly have tender extrathoracic adenopathy, fever, and weight loss. As stated earlier, intrathoracic adenopathy is the rule, with both hilar and mediastinal involvement (Pastores, Nardich, Aranda, McGuiness, & Rom, 1993). The adenopathy tends to be massive, presenting as extensive, heterogenous soft tissue lesions, presumably due to coalescence of matted nodes. In most reported series, right-sided paratracheal and mediastinal involvement is commonly noted. The finding of a ring-enhancing lesion on chest CT with multiple central areas of low attenuation after the injection of contrast material, rarely noted in other diseases, is very suggestive of the diagnosis of mediastinal tuberculosis.

The diagnosis of tuberculosis is usually made by needle aspiration or biopsy of the affected lymph node. In non–HIV-infected individuals there is a lower yield of acid-fast organisms on needle aspiration, roughly 25% to 50%, as compared to 67% to 90% in HIV-infected patients. However, as expected, the non–HIV-infected are more likely to show granuloma formation on biopsy. Therefore, an excisional node biopsy should be performed on all cases of suspected tuberculous adenitis if the results of needle aspiration are not diagnostic. Culture of lymph nodes provides a positive culture in greater than two thirds of cases.

Pleural Tuberculosis

Pleural tuberculosis is seen in approximately 20% of cases of extrapulmonary tuberculosis. Unlike lymphatic tuberculosis, the frequencies and clinical presentations in HIV- and non–HIV-infected individuals are very similar. In a recent series of hospitalized AIDS patients, effusions were attributed to tuberculosis in only 10% of cases (Joseph & Sahn, 1993). However, tuberculosis accounted for almost one third of effusions due to infection, and approximately one half of moderate to large effusions.

Pleural effusion in tuberculosis develops by two basic mechanisms. The most common is the development of a hypersensitivity reaction to a small number of organisms which reach the pleural space via direct spread or through subpleural lymphatics. As cell-mediated immunity progresses, a granulomatous reaction occurs in the pleura, but no organisms are seen on pleural biopsy. The patient may be asymptomatic or develop an acute syndrome with high fever. Fever, cough, and dull pleuritic pain over the location of the fluid are common clinical findings and occur in one half to two thirds of patients. If the effusion is large, dyspnea may also be present. The chest radiograph typically demonstrates a unilateral effusion, which is small to moderate in 80% of cases. A careful search for parenchymal abnormalities should be performed and may be found in a third of cases. The PPD may be helpful and is usually positive in non–HIV-infected patients. Examination of the pleural fluid demonstrates a serous, and occasionally serosanguinous, effusion. Biochemical analysis of the pleural fluid demonstrates an elevated protein and lactate dehydrogenase (LDH), consistent with an exudative effusion. The pleural fluid pH (less than 7.30) and glucose (less than 60 mg/dl) are decreased in only 20% of cases. The cell count generally shows less than 5,000 cells/ml, with a predominance of lymphocytes on differential counts. Despite generalized lymphopenia in HIV-infected patients, the pleural fluid in tuberculosis is characteristically lymphocyte rich. Interestingly, if there are greater than 10% eosinophils or greater than 5% mesothelial cells noted on pleural fluid differential cell count the diagnosis of tuberculosis is considered unlikely.

An immediate diagnosis is rarely established on acid-fast smears of pleural fluid, which are positive in less than 10% of cases. Although pleural fluid cultures have a higher yield (25%–35%), the diagnosis is delayed for several weeks. Pleural biopsy is the single best diagnostic study to perform in the evaluation of pleural tuberculosis. In non–HIV-infected individuals, a presumptive diagnosis is made by demonstrating a granuloma in 50% to 80% of cases. However, in the HIV-infected individual, granulomas may be less well formed, or only a lymphocytic infiltrate may be present on biopsy. Culture of pleural biopsy, like pleural fluid, has a high yield, and grows M. *tuberculosis* in 55% to 80% of cases. Furthermore, the combined yield of pleural fluid and pleural tissue histology and culture for tuberculosis proves the diagnosis in 70% to 85% of cases (Scharer & McClement, 1967).

The second, and fortunately less common, type of pleural involvement of tuberculosis is that of a frank empyema. There is a large inoculum of organisms introduced into the pleural space by either rupture of a cavity, or an adjacent parenchymal focus via a bronchopleural fistula. Unlike the patient with the hypersensitivity form of tuberculous effusion, the patient generally appears toxic and parenchymal involvement is usually evident on the chest radiograph.

Thoracentesis reveals a thick milky fluid, which is rich in fat or chyle. True chylous effusions contain high concentrations of triglycerides ($\geq$115 mg/dl). However, unlike chylous effusions, tuberculous empyemas are chyliform or made of "pseudo-chyle," and contain a high concentration of cholesterol with a normal to mildly increased amount of triglycerides. The fluid is exudative and usually has a high white blood count, which is predominately lymphocytic. Unlike the patients with the hypersensitivity form of pleural effusion, the acid-fast smears and mycobacterial cultures are usually positive, making pleural biopsy unnecessary.

Standard antituberculosis chemotherapy (discussed in chapter 5) is sufficient to successfully treat pleural tuberculosis. Thoracentesis is indicated only for drainage of symptomatic effusions. The long-term sequelae of pleural tuberculosis in most cases, given adequate chemotherapy, are generally minimal, with little to no pleural fibrosis. However, in patients with tuberculous empyema, who require both adequate chemotherapy and drainage, pleural fibrosis and calcification are common. Severe pleural fibrosis may decrease lung function and predispose to recurrent pneumonias.

The differential diagnosis of pleural tuberculosis includes infection due to bacteria, fungi, nocardia, atypical mycobacteria, and, rarely, *Pneumocystis carinii*. Of noninfectious causes, hypoalbuminemia and cardiac failure are most common, yet, because they are transudates and commonly bilateral, these entities are easily differentiated. However, both Kaposi's sarcoma and lymphoma may also present as moderate to large, lymphocyte-predominate exudates and pose the greatest diagnostic challenge.

Genitourinary Tuberculosis

Genitourinary tuberculosis, a relatively uncommon disorder, is seen in approximately 10% of patients with extrapulmonary tuberculosis. The kidneys are seeded during an initial bacillemia, and 90% of patients have bilateral lesions. However, most patients present with unilateral disease. Genital disease is likely to be spread from renal lesions, although hematogenous spread may also be the cause.

Local symptoms predominate, with dysuria, polyuria, hematuria, and flank pain. Common presentations have included recurrent urinary tract infection without growth of common bacterial pathogens, pyuria without bacteriuria, unexplained microscopic hematuria, and fever of unknown origin. Men may present a painless scrotal mass, a draining scrotal sinus, orchitis, prostatitis with induration, or epididymitis, particularly with calcification. Women may present with irregular menses, amenorrhea, pain secondary to pelvic inflammatory disease, or infertility.

The suspicion of genitourinary tuberculosis may be raised by chest radiographic evidence of old or active tuberculosis or a record of a positive PPD. An intravenous pyelogram, although nondiagnostic, may demonstrate multiple areas of abnormalities in the kidney and collecting system. Tuberculous involvement of the kidney causes destructive changes, including papillary necrosis, cavitation, and later calcification. The collecting system may demonstrate irregular calices, ureteral strictures, hydronephrosis, and contracture of the bladder. Rarely, renal function is significantly impaired. However, renal failure can occur if pre-existing renal disease is present. Furthermore, significant distortion of the collecting system may lead to recurrent bacterial infections and the development of nephrolithiasis. A diagnosis is generally obtained with repeat cultures of first-voided early morning urine specimens or is made on the basis of culture and histology of biopsy material. Diagnosis of genital lesions usually requires biopsy, because the differential diagnosis includes neoplasia as well as other infectious processes. Urine culture is the gold standard in the diagnosis of genitourinary tuberculosis, yielding a diagnosis in 80% to 90% of patients. Because positive urine cultures have been found in a significant proportion (20%) of patients with other forms of extrapulmonary tuberculosis without obvious genitourinary involvement, some clinicians recommend routine urine cultures in the work-up of suspected extrapulmonary tuberculosis.

Gastrointestinal Tuberculosis

Gastrointestinal tuberculosis is an uncommon manifestation of extrapulmonary tuberculosis, occurring in less than 5% of cases. Similarly, infections of the alimentary tracts of AIDS patients are rarely due to *M. tuberculosis*. However, *M. avium-intracellulare*, the most common cause of systemic bacterial infection in HIV-infected persons, is commonly associated with gastrointestinal symptoms. As stated earlier, stool cultures from HIV-infected patients which grow *M. tuberculosis* are more likely to be associated with aspirated pulmonary pathogens than to reflect primary intestinal disease.

Although uncommon, tuberculosis may involve any intra-abdominal organ as well as the peritoneum. After seeding from bacteremic spread, clinical disease is established by direct or late progression of infection. Peritonitis, the most common form of gastrointestinal tuberculosis, may develop from rupture of intra-abdominal lymph nodes and subsequent seeding of bacilli into the peritoneal cavity. As expected, the clinical manifestations of gastrointestinal tuberculosis depend on the localization and severity of infection.

Tuberculous peritonitis is often of insidious onset and difficult to diagnose. Before the current AIDS epidemic, the incidence of tuberculous peritonitis was estimated to be 0.1%–0.7% of all tuberculosis cases (Dineen, Homan, & Grafe, 1976). Tuberculous peritonitis in a patient with HIV infection is still fairly rare (Soubani & Glatt, 1992). The patient frequently presents with abdominal pain, distention, and fever. Weight loss and anorexia are also common. Physical examination may demonstrate ascites, a "doughy" abdomen, or an abdominal mass. The PPD has been variably reported to be positive (30%–100% of cases). The chest radiograph commonly shows pleural effusions, but lesions consistent with active tuberculosis are not commonly demonstrated. Computed tomographic scanning of the abdomen has been reported to show high density ascites with omental involvement and complex masses. The ascitic fluid is an exudate (>3 grams of protein per deciliter) with an elevated white blood cell count. Characteristically, there is a predominance of lymphocytes. However, early in the course of infection, polymorphonuclear cells may predominate. Like pleural fluid, acid-fast smears are rarely positive. Unfortunately, cultures of ascitic fluid grow tuberculosis in only one fourth to one half of cases, but the yield may be enhanced by culture of large volumes of fluid (>1 liter). Therefore, peritoneoscopy, culdoscopy, or laparotomy may be necessary to obtain biopsy material. This tissue is cultured for mycobacteria and may provide an immediate diagnosis by demonstrating granuloma. Peritoneoscopic biopsy has a reported efficacy of 85%, compared to the mini-laparotomy "gold standard."

Although intestinal involvement can be anywhere, it is rare to have disease proximal to the terminal ileum. Intestinal tuberculosis most commonly involves the terminal ileum and cecum, with other portions of the colon and the rectum involved less frequently. In the terminal ileum, the histology may reveal granulomatous inflammation with ulceration, and may be difficult to distinguished from Crohn's disease. In contrast, the cecum may demonstrate a proliferative form with luminal narrowing and the development of a mass. The presenting symptoms are nonspecific and include abdominal pain, anorexia, indigestion, constipation, or diarrhea. Barium studies of the bowel may demonstrate spasm, hypermotility of the bowel, or filling defects. Clinically, ileal involvement may suggest appendicitis, bowel obstruction, or Crohn's disease, while cecal involvement with tuberculosis is most commonly confused with carcinoma.

Tuberculous involvement of the rectum is usually in the form of anal fissures and perirectal abscesses. These lesions are generally quite painful and are associated with persistent drainage, causing patients to seek early medical attention.

Direct involvement of the esophagus is uncommon. It may be compressed by massively enlarged mediastinal lymph nodes. Occasionally, infection in mediastinal nodes may progress and cause localized inflammatory changes in the esophageal wall leading to strictures, perforations, and esophageal diverticula. Patients with strictures and diverticuli are at increased risk of aspiration pneumonia. Clinically, patients may present with dysphagia, chest pain, and cough and fever.

Tuberculous hepatitis has been considered a common complication of miliary tuberculosis. However, it is rarely found as an isolated entity, and clinically apparent hepatic involvement is rare. It is commonly associated with fever without jaundice, and hepatomegaly is not consistently found. The liver chemistries may demonstrate an infiltrative pattern with elevation of alkaline phosphatase and gamma-glutaryl transferase, yet normal bilirubin, SGOT, and serum glutamic pyruvate transaminase (SGPT; now known as alanine aminotransferase [ALT]). Rarely, abdominal radiographs will demonstrate hepatic calcifications. The diagnosis is established by liver biopsy showing a granulomatous hepatitis. It should be noted that the development of jaundice, hepatomegaly or liver chemistry abnormalities after the onset of therapy are more likely due to drug toxicity or hypersensitivity than tuberculous hepatitis.

In patients with AIDS, granulomatous hepatitis raises the possibility of drug toxicity or infection from fungi or mycobacteria. Mycobacteria, especially *M. avium-intracellulare,* are responsible for more than 90% of the specific diagnoses made by liver biopsy. Histology frequently reveals foci of histiocytes organized into poorly formed granuloma. More commonly in infections with *M. avium-intracellulare* than *M. tuberculosis,* stains for acid-fast bacilli are positive. Therefore, final determination of the pathogen requires bacteriologic isolation.

Splenic tuberculosis may be suspected when splenic calcification is noted on routine chest radiographs. However, rare cases of painful splenomegaly and splenic abscesses due to tuberculosis have been reported.

Skeletal Tuberculosis

Tuberculosis of the long bones, vertebrae, and joint spaces are uncommon forms of extrapulmonary tuberculosis in both HIV- and non–HIV-infected adult patients. Children and the elderly are most commonly affected. In the child, the epiphyseal growth plates are optimal sites for seeding during the initial bacillemia, presumably due to their increased vascularity, high oxygen tension, and a paucity of phagocytic cells. The organisms may also gain access to the vertebra from the pleural and paravertebral lymphatics. In these locations, the bacilli may lie dormant for several years until trauma or immunosuppression induce reactivation of the infection. Infection may then spread from the subchondral bone region to the synovium, cartilage, and joint space, leading to metaphyseal erosions and cysts, cartilage destruction, and joint space narrowing. Occasionally, infected material may escape the joint space and induce a paravertebral or periarticular abscess, which may develop a sinus tract to the skin.

Tuberculous arthritis, a sequela of adjacent osteomyelitis, commonly occurs in a single large weight-bearing joint; like osseous tuberculosis, it may also be multifocal. Tuberculous osteomyelitis may involve any bone; however, vertebral infection, or Pott's disease of the spine, is the most common form of osseous infection. The lumbar and upper thoracic spine is most commonly affected in adults, whereas the upper thoracic spine is commonly involved in children. The hips and knees are the most likely long bones affected, followed by the shoulders, elbows, ankles and wrist bones.

The presentation is usually indolent. Pain may be present for several months before x-rays demonstrate a change. Physical exam may reveal focal tenderness, swelling, and, rarely, sinus tracts. Delayed diagnosis may lead to bony deformities in children, or a catastrophic presentation with acute paraplegia from cord compression. The chest film may demonstrate evidence of old or active tuberculosis in one half of cases. Pleural effusions or a paravertebral mass may be the only diagnostic clues. The bone radiographs are not specific for tuberculosis, and initially, may only demonstrate soft tissue swelling, subchondral bone loss and cysts. Later, sclerosis, joint space narrowing and periarticular collections may be found. Given the poor sensitivity of plain films, computed tomographic scans should be performed of suspected vertebral lesions. Magnetic resonance imaging may be particularly helpful in cases where cord compression is suspected. Similarly, radionuclide bone and gallium scanning may be useful in defining both clinically suspected and unsuspected areas that lack radiographic abnormalities.

Isolation of tuberculous organisms or demonstration of granulomatous inflammation in the absence of an alternative explanation is sufficient to make the diagnosis. Joint fluid may demonstrate acid-fast organisms in up to a fourth of cases, with cultures growing tuberculous organisms in three fourths. In the absence of joint fluid, or periarticular abscesses, both bone and synovial biopsies may be performed, with high diagnostic yields.

Pericardial Tuberculosis

Although an uncommon complication of tuberculosis in both HIV- and non–HIV-infected patients, pericarditis is potentially fatal and requires early recognition and treatment. Both an acute form and chronic calcific pericarditis have been described; however, the latter form is very rare in HIV-infected patients.

The pericardium may be seeded with organisms during the initial bacillemia, bacillemia after reactivation, or, most commonly, from direct extension of disease from adjacent tissues. The lung parenchyma, pleura or tracheobronchial lymph nodes are the most likely foci of infection, and usually transmit a small inoculum of bacilli to the pericardium. As in pleural tuberculosis, a hypersensitivity reaction to mycobacterial antigens ensues with the development of a fibrinous or serofibrinous serositis. In rare instances, rupture of a caseous lymph node or cavity may introduce a large inoculum of bacilli into the pericardium and lead to a purulent form of pericarditis. These patients tend to present more acutely, with more clinical symptoms and rapid hemodynamic deterioration. Most patients with pericardial tuberculosis, however, have an insidious onset of symptoms with slow accumulation of pericardial fluid. In these instances, the pericardium may expand to accommodate large volumes of fluid (2 to 4 liters) with few hemodynamic sequelae.

The clinical presentation is not specific for tuberculosis. Symptoms of acute pericarditis with pleuritic precordial chest pain, which may be relieved with sitting up or leaning forward, are not consistently found in tuberculous pericarditis. Dyspnea, orthopnea, cough, and edema usually occur late, when a large effusion is present. However, constitutional symptoms of fever, night sweats, weight loss, and fatigue are commonly observed.

The physical examination may demonstrate a pericardial friction rub, which may have presystolic, systolic, or early diastolic scratchy components, best appreciated during inspiration, with the patient upright and leaning forward. Clinical findings of tachycardia, tachypnea, low blood pressure, pulsus paradoxus, jugular venous distention, hepatomegaly, and edema should be sought, and may suggest the development of cardiac tamponade.

As expected, the laboratory studies are nonspecific. The chest radiograph will show an enlarged cardiac silhouette in the acute form, frequently without evidence for pulmonary tuberculosis. However, the presence of a chronic pericardial effusion and a positive PPD should heighten the clinical suspicion for tuberculosis. The pericardial fluid is exudative with an elevated total protein and LDH. The white blood cell count is generally less than 10,000/mm^3, and shows a predominance of mononuclear cells. As in pleural fluid, direct smears are rarely positive and cultures grow tuberculosis in up to 30% of cases. Pericardial biopsy for both histologic and bacteriologic evaluation is frequently required to effectively diagnose and treat pericardial tuberculosis. In instances where pericardial biopsy is inconclusive and there remains a high clinical suspicion, antituberculous therapy should be provided given the high mortality (approximately 70%) of untreated symptomatic disease.

In patients who develop a subacute illness, chronic inflammation with thickening of the pericardium and epicardium may occur, leading to varying amounts of loculated fluid and pericardial fibrosis, which may lead to impaired filling of the cardiac chambers. The patients demonstrate signs of low cardiac output, predominately right heart failure and proteinuria, consistent with constrictive pericarditis. Radiographs may demonstrate a small heart with pericardial calcification, and up to 50% of patients have evidence of old or active tuberculosis. Cardiac catheterization and/or echocardiograms are commonly performed to physiologically confirm the presence of constrictive pericarditis. Total pericardiectomy is recommended to resolve the cardiovascular consequences.

Laryngeal Tuberculosis

This rare form of extrapulmonary tuberculosis requires special attention because of the highly infectious nature of patients with involvement of the larynx and adjacent structures. Frequently, laryngeal tuberculosis occurs in the setting of very advanced pulmonary tuberculosis. Large volumes of bacilli from expectorated sputum adhere to and invade the mucosa of the vocal cords, epiglottis, and hypopharynx. Initially, there is mild inflammation with erythema, edema, and ulceration of the cords. Later, extensive ulceration, scarring, distortion, and narrowing of the larynx and epiglottis may develop.

Clinically, the patients present with hoarseness, sore throat, and cough. As the disease progresses, severe dysphonia, dysphagia, throat pain, and dyspnea develop. Chest radiographs invariably show extensive pulmonary disease with cavitary lesions, and occasionally, bilateral alveolar infiltrates due to transbronchial spread. Diagnosis may be established by sputum smears and radiographic findings of laryngeal

TABLE 3.1 Some Reported Sites of Nonpulmonary Tuberculosis

Site	Syndrome
1. Eye	Chorioretinitis, iridocyclitis, iritis, granulomatous conjunctivitis
2. Ear	Chronic otitis media, mastoiditis
3. Throat	Tonsillitis, buccal mucosal ulcers
4. Chest wall	Draining sinus or "empyema necessitatus"
5. Mediastinum	Mediastinal fibrosis, Superior Vena Cava syndrome
6. Heart	Myocardial and endocardial infiltration
7. Vessels	Mycotic aneurysms, Rasmussen's aneurysm of pulmonary vessels
8. Retroperitoneum	Retroperitoneal fibrosis, obstructive uropathy
9. Endocrine	Syndrome of inappropriate antidiuretic hormone (SIADH), adrenal cortical insufficiency (Addison's disease), hypercalcemia, sick euthyroid syndrome
10. Soft tissue	Abscesses
11. Breast	Mastitis
12. Skin	Ulcer, hypersensitivity vasculitis, erythema nodosum

and epiglottic edema on lateral neck radiographs. However, on occasion, direct laryngoscopy and biopsy may be required in mild cases, when cancer is considered in the differential diagnosis.

Other Organs

As stated earlier tuberculosis may affect any site at the time of hematogenous dissemination or by contiguous spread. Other reported sites and clinical syndromes are described in Table 3.1.

REFERENCES

Abernathy, R. S. (1987). Tuberculosis in children: Still a public health threat. *Journal of Respiratory Disease, 8*(2), 67–87.

American Thoracic Society. (1990). American Thoracic Society statement: Diagnostic standards and classification of tuberculosis. *American Review of Respiratory Disease, 142,* 725–735.

Berenguer, J., Moreno, S., Laguna, F., Vincente, T., Adrados, M., Ortega, A., Gonzalez-LaHoz, J., & Bouza, E. (1992). Tuberculous meningitis in patients infected with human immunodeficiency virus. *New England Journal of Medicine, 326,* 668–672.

Braun, M. M., Byers, R. H., Heynard, W. L., Ciesielski, C. A., Bloch, A. B., Berkelman, R. L., & Snider, D. E. (1990). Acquired immunodeficiency syndrome and extrapulmonary tuberculosis in the United States. *Archives of Internal Medicine, 150,* 1913–1916.

Dannenberg, A. M. (1993). Immunopathogenesis of pulmonary tuberculosis. *Hospital Practice, 28*(1), 51–58.

Dineen, P., Homan, W. P., & Grafe, W. R. (1976). Tuberculous peritonitis: 43 year experience in diagnosis and treatment. *Annals in Surgery, 184,* 717–722.

Good, J. T., Seman, M. D., Davidson, P. T., Lakshminarayan, S., & Sahn, S. A. (1981). Tuberculosis in association with pregnancy. *American Journal of Obstetrics and Gynecology, 140,* 492–498.

Heffner, J. E., Strange, C., & Sahn, S. A. (1988). The impact of respiratory failure on the diagnosis of tuberculosis. *Archives of Internal Medicine, 148,* 1103–1108.

Joseph, J., & Sahn, S. A. (1993). Pleural effusions in hospitalized patients with AIDS. *Annals of Internal Medicine, 118,* 856–859.

Keers, R. Y. (1978). Tuberculosis in antiquity. In *Tuberculosis: A journey down the centuries* (pp. 1–5). London: Bailleire Tindall.

Khouri, Y. F., Mastrucci, M. T., Hutto, C., Mitchell, C. D., & Scott, G. B. (1992). *Mycobacterium tuberculosis* in children with human immunodeficiency virus infection. *Pediatric Infectious Disease Journal, 11,* 950–955.

Kramer, F., Modilevsy, T., Waliant, A. R., Leedom, J. M., & Barnes, P. F. (1990). Delayed diagnosis of tuberculosis in patients with human immunodeficiency virus infection. *American Journal of Medicine, 89*(4), 451–456.

Modilevsky, T., Sattler, F. R., & Barnes, P. F. (1989). Mycobacterial disease in patients with human immunodeficiency virus infection. *Archives of Internal Medicine, 149,* 2201–2205.

Munt, P. W. (1971). Miliary tuberculosis in the chemotherapy era: With a clinical review in 69 American adults. *Medicine, 51*(2), 139–155.

Murray, J. F., & Mills, J. (1990). State of the art: Pulmonary infectious complications of human immunodeficiency virus infection, Part 1. *American Review of Respiratory Disease, 141,* 1356–1372.

New York City Department of Health. (1991). Tuberculosis in New York City: The 1990 experience. *City Health Information, 10*(2), 1–6.

Pastores, S. M., Nardich, D. P., Aranda, C. P., McGuiness, L., & Rom, W. N. (1993). Intrathoracic adenopathy associated with pulmonary tuberculosis in patients with human immunodeficiency virus infection. *Chest, 105,* 1433–1437.

Scharer, L., & McClement, J. H. (1967). Isolation of tubercle bacilli from needle biopsy specimens of parietal pleura. *American Review of Respiratory Disease, 97,* 466–468.

Shafer, R. W., Kim, D. S., Weiss, J. P., & Quale, J. M. (1991). Extrapulmonary tuberculosis in patients with human immunodeficiency virus infection. *Medicine, 70,* 384–397.

Soubani, A. O., & Glatt, A. E. (1992). Tuberculous peritonitis as an initial manifestation of HIV infection. *New York State Journal of Medicine, 92*(6), 269–270.

Theuer, C. P., Hopewell, P. C., Elias, D., Schecter, G. F., Rutherford, G. S., & Chaisson, R. E. (1990). Human immunodeficiency virus infection in tuberculosis patients. *Journal of Infectious Diseases, 162,* 8–12.

Turcios, N. L., & Evans, H. E. (1989). Establishing the diagnosis of tuberculosis in children. *Journal of Respiratory Diseases, 10*(5), 15–30.

Vallejo, J. G., & Starke, J. R. (1992). Tuberculosis and pregnancy. *Clinics in Chest Medicine, 13,* 693–707.

Yamaguchi, E., & Reichman, L. B. (1992). Tuberculosis and HIV: Keep a high index of suspicion! *Journal of Respiratory Diseases, 13,* 1301–1323.

4

Diagnosis of Tuberculous Infection and Disease

When we breathe air contaminated by an infectious patient with active pulmonary tuberculosis, we may become infected with the tubercle bacillus. Once infected, an individual may or may not go on to develop actual disease. It is estimated that in normal, immunocompetent hosts, about 5% will develop active disease in the first 2 years following infection and another 5% during their lifetimes.

The incidence of tuberculosis among patients with AIDS is almost 500 times the incidence in the general population (Pitchenik, Fertel, & Block, 1988). In addition, the risk of tuberculosis among HIV-infected individuals with positive tuberculin skin tests is very high, estimated to be 8% per year (Selwyn, Hartel, & Lewis, 1989). HIV infection clearly increases the risk of reactivation of latent tuberculous infection and promotes progressive disease from newly acquired infection (Daley, Small, & Schecter, 1992).

It is obviously important, therefore, to diagnose infection when it occurs in all potential patients, but especially in those with HIV infection. Screening in the United States is usually done in groups with a high risk of exposure to tuberculosis (e.g., close contacts of known infectious cases), but also in persons with other medical risk factors known to increase the risk of developing active tuberculosis, such as HIV infection.

In general, the purpose of screening is to identify infected individuals who would benefit from preventive therapy. In chapter 5 we will review current guidelines for such therapy. This chapter includes current guidelines concerning screening by demographic criteria, and outlines those medical conditions that increase the risk of developing clinical tuberculosis once infection has occurred.

First we will describe the available methods of screening for infection with the tubercle bacillus and review the current classification of positive reactions.

TUBERCULIN SKIN TESTING

In chapter 2 on pathogenesis, we reviewed the development of delayed hypersensitivity to the tuberculin protein. It has been known for over 100 years that 2 to 10 weeks following infection an individual will usually develop a positive skin test to protein derived from the tubercle bacillus. Soon after he discovered the tubercle bacillus, Robert Koch prepared a concentrated extract which he called *old tuberculin* (OT), which he thought would be useful in the treatment of the disease. After a few years, OT proved useless as a treatment, but this crude extract contained a number of antigens which provoked a reaction in the skin of people with tuberculosis. It has taken many years to standardize the skin testing material and to formalize the proper way to perform the test to detect people infected with the tubercle bacillus.

In the 1930s, Florence Seibert developed a purified protein derivative of OT which is now called PPD-S and is currently the standard reference material in the United States. Her compound initially was available as a tablet or powder which had to be reconstituted with a dilutent, but in subsequent years it could be made in liquid form by the addition of a detergent (Tween), which prevents its absorption by glass or plastic containers and syringes.

It is now generally agreed that the Mantoux method, an intracutaneous injection of a standard undiluted antigen, is the method of choice. Because the Mantoux test takes more time and expertise to administer, however, many physicians and nurses have preferred to use a multiple-puncture test such as the tine test, especially when screening young children. The Mantoux method is clearly superior and should always be used when screening for tuberculous infection. Multiple-puncture tests, although quick and convenient, have many potential problems, including loss of antigen from the prongs of the disc, lack of standardization of the antigen dose, variability in the application of the prongs (too shallow or too deep), and lack of standardization in test reading.

Technique

The Mantoux test is performed by the intradermal injection of 0.1 ml of PPD tuberculin containing 5 tuberculin units (TU) into the volar or dorsal surface of the forearm. The injection, which should be made with a disposable tuberculin syringe with a short 26- or 27-gauge needle, is placed just beneath the surface of the skin with the needle bevel facing upward to produce a discrete elevation of the skin (a wheal) 6 to 10 mm in diameter.

Significant or Positive Reactions

The skin test should be read 48 to 72 hours after the injection. Positive reactions often remain as long as one week after the injection. The measurement of induration, not erythema, determines a positive reaction; it should be recorded in millimeters.

Biopsies of tuberculin reactions show accumulations of polymorphonuclear cells followed by lymphocytes and macrophages. Vascular leakage of plasma proteins and the subsequent formation of an intradermal fibrin clot accounts for most of the induration. This entire reaction is dependent on functioning CD4+ cells.

For many years the standard positive reaction was any induration over 10 mm, but in 1990 the "Diagnostic Standards and Classification of Tuberculosis" (American Thoracic Society, 1990) were revised to include three separate size reactions based on risk factors for disease and likelihood of true infection with M. *tuberculosis*. These new guidelines are listed in Table 4.1.

A tuberculin reaction of 5 mm or more is considered positive in persons with known or suspected HIV infection, persons with close and

TABLE 4.1 Criteria for Classification of Purified Protein Derivative (PPD) Skin Tests as Significant

Induration in mm	Social and/or medical conditions
5–9	HIV infection
	Major risk factor for HIV infection
	Recent contact with infectious case of tuberculosis
	Abnormal chest x-ray consistent with old healed tuberculosis
10–14	Intravenous drug users known to be HIV negative
	Risk factors for tuberculosis, including silicosis, gastrectomy, chronic renal failure, diabetes mellitus, prolonged immunosuppressive therapy
	Foreign-born persons from countries with a high prevalence of tuberculosis
	Medically underserved, low-income populations
	Residents of long-term-care facilities, including jails and nursing homes
≥15	Members of low-incidence tuberculosis groups without the risk factors listed above

Source: Centers for Disease Control. (1991, April). *Core Curriculum on Tuberculosis* (2nd ed.). Publication of the National Tuberculosis Training Initiative of the Centers for Disease Control and the American Thoracic Society, Atlanta.

recent contact with a patient with active tuberculosis, and persons with abnormal chest x-rays suggesting old, healed tuberculosis.

A tuberculin reaction of 10 mm or more is considered positive in individuals with medical conditions that increase the risk of developing tuberculosis once infection has occurred. These include the conditions listed above plus diabetes mellitus, silicosis, end-stage renal disease, chronic malabsorption syndromes, and prolonged corticosteroid therapy or any other condition which causes immunosuppression. Furthermore, 10-mm reactions are considered positive in foreign-born persons from high-prevalence countries, low-income populations, including high-risk minorities (especially blacks, Hispanics, and Native Americans), intravenous drug users, and residents of long-term-care facilities such as jails and nursing homes.

A tuberculin reaction of 15 mm or more is considered positive in all other individuals without the risk factors described above. These positive reactors have no known exposure to tuberculosis and reactions in this group between 5 and 15 mm are thought to represent cross-reactions to nontuberculous mycobacteria, as well as some with true tuberculous exposure.

The standard test dose of commercially available PPD is defined as the dose of the product that is biologically equivalent to 5 TU of PPD-S; the dose should cause reactions of equivalent size. Also available are products labeled 1 TU and 250 TU, but they are not bioassayed. They contain one fifth and 50 times the concentration of antigen in 5 TU. Some workers in the field have used 1 TU when they feared a very large reaction based on past history. A positive reaction would still be from 5 to 15 mm as defined above. Most testers, however, would only use the routine 5 TU dose for routine screening. The 250 TU product has been used as a nonspecific antigen in assessing a patient's immunologic status, but it obviously should never be used without being sure that there is no reaction to 5 TU. A positive reaction does not mean the same as a positive reaction to 5 TU. Occasionally a very sensitive individual will react to 5 TU with a vesicular or ulcerating local reaction, rarely including lymphangitis, regional adenopathy and fever. Keeping the reaction clean to prevent secondary infection is all the treatment necessary. Some have used topical corticosteroids, applied with an occlusive plastic dressing, before the full reaction develops, but it is not proven that this works. Skin testing does not cause delayed hypersensitivity to develop, but may have a booster effect, as described later in this chapter. Many years ago it was feared that testing a patient with inactive tuberculosis might lead to a systemic reaction and activation of disease but there is no proof that this occurs and with current drug therapy this is not a consideration.

False-Negative Reactions

Unfortunately, the absence of a reaction to the tuberculin skin test does not exclude the diagnosis of tuberculosis. Causes of false-negative reactions are listed in Table 4.2. There are many well-known situations and illnesses which interfere with cell-mediated immunity, the best known

TABLE 4.2 Causes of a False-Negative Tuberculin Skin Test

1. Concurrent illness
   HIV infection
   Immunosuppressive diseases
   Severe febrile illness
   Overwhelming tuberculosis (e.g., miliary)
   Acute viral infections (e.g., measles, mumps, etc.)
   Renal failure
   Malnutrition
   Sarcoidosis
   Immunosuppressive drugs (e.g., corticosteroids, etc.)

2. Testing procedure problems
   Subcutaneous injection
   Improper storage of PPD
   Delayed injection after filling syringe
   Lack of experience in interpretation

being HIV infection, and lead to a negative skin test. Others include any severe or febrile illness, measles and other exanthemas, Hodgkin's disease, overwhelming miliary or pulmonary tuberculosis, sarcoidosis, and the use of corticosteroids or other immunosuppressive drugs.

Factors related to the testing procedure that may cause a false-negative tuberculin reaction include subcutaneous injection, improper storage of the PPD, and lack of experience in interpretation.

Up to 30% of individuals without HIV infection may have skin test reactions less than 5 mm even though they are infected with tubercle bacilli. It is unfortunate that we must rely on a test with such a potential for false-negative reactions, but at present it is the only test available to diagnose tuberculous infection. When tuberculosis becomes an active disease we have many other options as will be discussed below.

If HIV infection is present, especially with progression to AIDS, the chance of a negative reaction (less than 5 mm induration) with known tuberculous infection is as high as 60%. Some have even suggested using 2 mm as a positive reaction in this group, but for the present 5 mm is the standard cut-off.

Tuberculin skin testing should be done at least annually on HIV-infected persons who are skin-test negative on the initial evaluation even though the CD4+ lymphocyte count may fall during this time period. If conversion occurs then not only have we documented tuberculous infection but also alerted health care workers to the possibility of an infectious case in the environment and the need to look for a possible source case.

Anergy Testing

The CDC has published guidelines for anergy testing and management of anergic persons at risk of tuberculosis (CDC, 1991) (see Table 4.3). They point out that studies of tuberculous disease associated with HIV infection show that a large number of patients will have PPD anergy if their tuberculosis is concurrent with other HIV-related infections. In various studies the mean CD4 count for PPD-positive (greater than 5 mm reaction) was 220 per mm^3 compared with 66 per mm^3 for PPD-negative patients.

TABLE 4.3 Summary of Guidelines for Anergy Testing

1. All persons with HIV infection should receive a PPD-tuberculin skin test (5TU, PPD by Mantoux method).

2. Because of the occurrence of anergy to PPD among persons with HIV infection at risk of tuberculosis, persons with HIV infection should also be evaluated for DTH anergy at the time of PPD testing.

3. Companion testing with two DTH antigens (*Candida,* mumps, or tetanus toxoid) administered by the Mantoux method is recommended. However, a multipuncture device which administers a battery of DTH antigens may be used.

4. Any induration to a DTH antigen measured at 48 hours to 72 hours is considered evidence of DTH responsiveness; failure to elicit a response is considered evidence of anergy.

5. Those persons with a positive (≥5 mm induration) PPD reaction are considered to be infected with *M. tuberculosis* and should be evaluated for isoniazid preventive therapy after active tuberculosis has been excluded.

6. Persons who manifest a DTH response but, have a negative PPD reaction are, in general, considered not to be infected with *M. tuberculosis.*

7. Anergic, tuberculin-negative persons whose risk of tuberculous infection is estimated to be ≥10% should also be considered for isoniazid preventive therapy after active tuberculosis is excluded.

8. Although CD4 counts should be performed as a part of the evaluation and management of persons with HIV infection, this measurement is not a substitute for anergy evaluation.

Source: Centers for Disease Control. (1991). Purified protein derivative (PPD)-Tuberculin anergy and HIV infection: Guidelines for anergy testing and management of anergic persons at risk of tuberculosis. *Morbidity and Mortality Weekly Report, 40,* (RR-5), 27–33.

Because of the chance of PPD anergy in asymptomatic persons with HIV infection, delayed type hypersensitivity (DTH) testing with two other skin test antigens (e.g., candida, mumps, or tetanus toxoid) should be done at the same time as PPD testing. This is based on the assumption that most healthy people would be sensitive to one of these antigens. At present mumps antigen is the only one standardized for this purpose, but the others can be used as well. A reaction greater than 2 mm of induration to any of these is considered positive. A multiple-puncture device is available that delivers seven different DTH antigens percutaneously, but this method is not as accurate as DTH antigens administered by the Mantoux method (e.g., 0.1 ml intradermally).

If an individual has a positive response to one or more of these other DTH antigens and not to tuberculin (PPD), he or she is not considered to be infected with *M. tuberculosis*. However, a negative PPD reaction, even with a positive reaction to other DTH antigens, should never be used to exclude the diagnosis of active tuberculosis. As noted earlier there are numerous technical and/or biological reasons for a false negative skin test. Furthermore, Blatt et al. (1993), using four control skin test antigens (mumps, candida, tetanus toxoid, and trichophyton) showed that response to one skin test only (using a definition of a positive result requiring at least 5 mm of induration) correlates with significant immunosuppression. They suggested that individuals with this "partial anergy" may still be at risk for false-negative tuberculin skin test results despite tuberculous infection.

The Booster Effect

Once hypersensitivity to tuberculin develops, the skin test reaction may slowly wane over many years so that a standard 5 TU tuberculin skin test may be negative (Thompson, Glassroth, Snider, & Farer, 1979). The skin test may recall or stimulate hypersensitivity so that another test after one week or one year will now be positive. This is not a conversion of the skin test from negative to positive, but simply a "boosted" reaction, and most commonly seen in individuals over 55 years. Many health care facilities that care for patients with tuberculosis will do a second skin test, using 5 TU, on employees who are PPD negative on employment, following the procedure described in Table 4.4. In this group, who will be undergoing periodic PPD skin testing, it is impor-

TABLE 4.4 Two-Step Tuberculin Skin Testing

1. Perform PPD testing in the usual manner with 0.1 ml of 5 tuberculin units (5 TU).
2. If the reaction to the first test is negative, give a second test with the same dose and strength of tuberculin 1–3 weeks later. (If the first test was positive, the individual is classified as infected and there is no need for second test.)
3. If the second test is positive, the person is classified as infected.
4. If the second test is negative, the person is classified as uninfected.
5. All individuals who have a positive reaction to either test require a follow-up evaluation and chest x-ray.

Source: Modified from New York City Department of Health. (1993). *Tuberculosis at a Glance.*

tant to know if their initial test is definitely negative or positive. If the second test is done one or two weeks after the first, a positive reaction is clearly from the booster effect and not secondary to infection acquired while working in the facility.

Repeated skin testing will not cause a positive reaction to develop unless the test is always administered in the same exact location.

If an individual gives a history of vaccination with BCG or is from a foreign country where it is commonly used, a positive tuberculin test (a reaction of 10 mm or more of induration) may be from the vaccination or from infection with *M. tuberculosis*. Since conversion rates after BCG vaccination are not 100% and the mean reaction size is often less than 10 mm, most experts in the field recommend that the positive test be treated as a new infection or from infection acquired in the country where the BCG was given, but each case must be individually evaluated.

HISTORY AND PHYSICAL EXAMINATION

In chapter 3 on clinical presentation, the usual history and physical examination of patients with active tuberculosis is discussed.

RADIOLOGY

Once there is a clinical suspicion of tuberculosis, one of the most common and useful tests is a chest x-ray. Although no radiographic appearance is unique to tuberculosis, certain patterns are well known to occur. In patients with HIV infection the same is true, but we see a greater variety of changes depending on the extent of immune system compromise. These patterns are discussed in chapter 3.

SPUTUM, BLOOD, URINE, AND
TISSUE SPECIMENS

Smears for Acid-Fast Bacilli

Once there is a clinical suspicion of active disease, the first step is to confirm the diagnosis by isolation of the infecting organism, *Mycobacterium tuberculosis*. From the time of its discovery it has been known as "acid-fast" because of its resistance, once stained, to decolorization with acid alcohol. The presence of acid-fast organisms in a specimen is suggestive of the diagnosis but until the organism is actually cultured, there is not actual proof. Since tuberculosis can occur in many possible sites, various specimens can be submitted to the laboratory to look for acid-fast bacilli (AFB) in stained smears examined under the microscope, but the same material must also be cultured to try and grow the organism. There are various techniques available to stain for AFB. The most traditional has been the Ziehl-Neelsen method, in which the bacillus appears as a small straight red or pink rod against a blue background (if methylene blue is used as a counterstain). Most laboratories now use a fluorescent staining method with fluorochrome, which makes slides easier to scan but is more nonspecific.

Polymerase Chain Reaction

New technology has been developed called the *polymerase chain reaction* (PCR), which amplifies specific DNA sequences for direct detection of the organism at the molecular level in 2 days. In theory, PCR is capable of detecting a single organism in a specimen such as blood, sputum, lavage fluid, pleural fluid, or cerebrospinal fluid (Eisenstein, 1990). At present the test is expensive and not proven in clinical trials as being better than standard stains in sputum testing. Its potential use at present is in smear-negative cases as well as for early diagnosis in extrapulmonary cases, especially tuberculous meningitis. Culture must still be done to confirm the diagnosis and provide antimicrobial susceptibility.

Since pulmonary tuberculosis is the most common form of tuberculosis, sputum specimens are the most commonly submitted material for smear and culture. Usually three early morning specimens collected on successive days are all that is necessary but if these are negative on smear, then three more specimens should be submitted. Levy et al. reported a sensitivity of 53.1% and a specificity of 99.8% for sputum smears. For both smear and culture, 95% of their positive results were obtained by examining three sputum samples (Levy et al., 1989). Other series have shown similar results, with a range depending on clinical presentation. Kim, Blackman, and Heatwole (1984) found that 74.4% (727 of 977) patients with pulmonary tuberculosis had positive sputum smears. Another group (Greenbaum, Beyt, & Murray, 1980) reported positive smears in 52% of patients with cavitary disease, but only 32% with local infiltrates.

There is no advantage to a 24-hour collection over a single morning specimen. The larger specimens are prone to contamination by other organisms. Often the patient must be instructed on how to produce a good specimen and not to be satisfied with just saliva. If the patient is unable to raise sputum, then sputum can be induced using various aerosol mists.

Other methods have been used in the past to obtain material for culture of tubercle bacilli. These include a laryngeal swab (where a moist sterile cotton swab is touched on the larynx to stimulate coughing and droplets adhering to the cotton can be cultured), transnasal or transtracheal aspiration, and even tracheal lavage. Because these methods produce a vigorous cough, they pose the risk of contamination of the air by tubercle bacilli and potential spread of disease.

Bronchoscopy

Since active tuberculosis can be more life-threatening in patients with HIV infection and AIDS, finding sputum positive for AFB can lead to an earlier presumptive diagnosis than waiting for a positive sputum culture. Studies have shown that more patients with AIDS and active pulmonary tuberculosis have negative AFB smears than non–HIV-infected patients with active tuberculosis (Klein et al., 1989). As seen earlier, this is probably due to the atypical presentation of pulmonary tuberculosis in AIDS patients (that is, fewer cavities and more infiltrative disease).

Where sputum is available and negative on smear for AFB, or simply cannot be obtained, then bronchoscopy may be indicated to make a more rapid diagnosis by providing additional material for study, including washings, brushings, and even biopsy specimens. There has been a steady increase in the use of this procedure to speed up obtaining material for AFB smear and culture when sputum is not quickly obtained. Bronchoscopy has been especially effective in patients with HIV infection, but also in the elderly when no sputum can be obtained (Patel et al., 1993).

As discussed earlier in chapter 3, the frequency of positive smears of both sputum and broncho-alveolar lavage varies greatly (30%–80%) depending on the clinical presentation and immune status of HIV-infected patients. In severely immunocompromised patients with active tuberculosis, the yield of these procedures may significantly decrease. In one group with initially negative sputum smears, bronchoscopy with lavage and transbronchial lung biopsy made an immediate diagnosis in roughly one third of the cases (Kennedy, Lewis, & Barnes, 1992). They made an immediate diagnosis of tuberculosis for 25 of 66 patients (38%) who had a negative sputum examination before bronchoscopy. There was no significant difference in the yield between HIV-infected and non–HIV-infected patients. Most of the increase in diagnosis was due to finding of granuloma on the lung biopsy specimen. The addition of biopsy to the procedure adds risks but clearly is necessary to increase the yield in rapid diagnoses.

Gastric Aspiration

Aspiration of fasting gastric contents can be done to obtain bronchial secretions that are swallowed while the patient is sleeping, but it is a laborious, invasive, and uncomfortable procedure. It is most useful in hospitalized patients and is done before they get out of bed in the morning. Aspiration is less likely to produce positive results in ambulatory patients because activity stimulates gastric activity and emptying of stomach contents. Although it is still used in children, the material obtained cannot be used for direct smears since there are nonpathogenic acid-fast organisms commonly present.

In HIV-infected patients with tuberculosis, stools are positive for acid-fast bacilli in 40% of patients. These patients rarely have evidence of gastrointestinal tuberculosis, so the finding of M. *tuberculosis* in stool culture usually represents organisms in swallowed sputum (Barnes, Bloch, Davidson, & Snider, 1991).

Isolator Blood Cultures

Mycobacterium tuberculosis bacteremia was reported in patients in the prechemotherapy era (Clough, 1917), but, until recently, blood cultures for mycobacteria were rarely performed. With the onset of the AIDS epidemic and disseminated tuberculosis, the test has become popular but is not indicated in all patients. Shafer, Goldberg, Siera, and Glatt (1989) found that 9 out of 59 patients with tuberculosis (15%) had positive blood cultures for M. *tuberculosis*. All the patients were HIV-infected, or had major risk factors for HIV infection. Admission sputum AFB smears were negative in all these patients. Again, all the patients had significant immunodeficiency, high fever, and clinical evidence of multiorgan tuberculous involvement (e.g., miliary infiltrates on chest x-ray). In all cases tuberculosis was diagnosed from some other site, so the blood cultures were not helpful in making the diagnosis, but the authors suggest that positive blood cultures may help confirm the diagnosis, especially when empiric therapy is necessary.

Most hospitals use a lysis-centrifugation system for culturing blood for mycobacteria. Blood cells are placed in a tube containing a lysing mixture in which they release mycobacteria. The mycobacteria are centrifuged and inoculated into culture media and then incubated. One blood culture system (BACTEC) has a specific medium designed for the recovery of mycobacteria from blood using a radioactive substrate, which is more expensive. In both cases it takes on the average of 3 weeks (range: 1–7 weeks) to grow the organism.

When nonpulmonary tuberculosis is suspected, other specimens can be submitted for examination, including urine, pleural fluid, pus, cerebrospinal fluid, bone marrow, and any biopsy specimen. Tissue specimens for culture of M. *tuberculosis* must be put into saline or special liquid medium and not formalin, which will kill the organism. Bone marrow and liver biopsy specimens are commonly used, but any material removed (lymph node biopsy, pleural biopsy, etc.) should be submitted for culture of tuberculosis if this diagnosis is under consideration.

Most clinical specimens (sputum, gastric aspiration, urine) are not collected in sterile containers, and are contaminated with more rapidly growing organisms. They must be decontaminated before culture is done. This is a standard procedure in all laboratories, but adds to the time it takes (usually 6–8 weeks) to grow M. *tuberculosis*. If the specimen comes from a sterile area (e.g., bone marrow aspiration or liver biopsy), then it must be collected in a sterile container and does not need decontamination procedures.

Culture of *Mycobacterium tuberculosis*

Culture of the organism remains the "gold standard" in making a definite diagnosis. Various culture media are available. The standard egg-based media (Jensen-Lowenstein), which is usually placed in screw-capped tubes, is the least expensive and supports colonies of organisms, but take the longest to show growth. Clear agar media, for example, 7H10, are usually placed in Petri dishes. Organisms are detected more quickly, but require special features such as a CO_2-enriched atmosphere, which make them more expensive. The quickest way to allow detection, but the most expensive, is the BACTEC-TB system, which measures carbon dioxide produced by the growth of tubercle bacilli in a liquid medium (Middlebrook, Reggiardo, & Tiggertt, 1977). Any of these three can also be used for drug susceptibility testing.

Because there is a delay in proving the diagnosis, treatment must be started when there are sufficient facts to suggest the diagnosis of tuberculosis, with enough drugs to cover various resistance possibilities. This practice is specific to tuberculosis, since most other bacteria provide culture and sensitivity information in 48 to 72 hours.

HISTOLOGY

Tuberculous Granuloma

Numerous biopsy procedures are available to confirm the diagnosis of tuberculosis. Whatever the specimen, the classic finding is the presence of tuberculous granuloma, usually with tubercle bacilli seen with special stains. Whether looking at lung, lymph node, liver, or any other body tissue, this basic lesion consisting of epithelioid cells and lymphocytes in a nodular shape with the usual addition of caseation and giant cells should be formed as the normal response by the host to infection by *M. tuberculosis*. The formation of poor granuloma or total absence was noted early in the study of patients with HIV infection by Sunderam and colleagues (Sunderam et al., 1986). In 17 patients with various biopsies, 8 had necrotizing granulomas, 6 had nonnecrotizing granulomas, and three did not reveal granulomas, although tubercle bacilli were cultured. Among the granuloma there was marked variation, from fully formed granuloma to barely recognizable aggregates.

Others have shown that granuloma formation is usually present in HIV-infected patients with tuberculosis, despite severe immunodeficiency (Jones et al., 1993). They speculate that granuloma formation is controlled by factors independent of the CD4 cell, such as tumor necrosis factor, which is released by macrophages.

In addition to material for the pathologist, clinicians should also obtain material for culture from a sterile area so that decontamination is not necessary. The opportunity to provide material for culture is important because the finding of granuloma formation is nonspecific and may occur in other diseases.

With hematogenous spread of tuberculosis, the yield of liver, bone marrow, and transbronchial lung biopsies for both histology and culture has been quite high, often when routine sputum and/or urine cultures are negative. Pleural biopsies are a standard diagnostic technique in patients suspected of tuberculous pleural effusions with high yields of histology and/or culture to confirm the diagnosis.

REFERENCES

American Thoracic Society. (1990). American Thoracic Society statement: Diagnostic standards and classification of tuberculosis. *American Review of Respiratory Disease, 142,* 725–735.

Barnes, P. F., Bloch, A. B., Davidson, P. T., & Snider, D. E., Jr. (1991).

Tuberculosis in patients with human immunodeficiency virus infection. *New England Journal of Medicine, 324,* 1644–1650.

Blatt, S. P., Hendrix, C. W., Butzin, C. A., Freeman, T. M., Ward, W. W., Hensley, R. E., Melcher, G. P., Donovan, D. J., & Boswell, R. N. (1993). Delayed-type hypersensitivity skin testing predicts progression to AIDS in HIV-infected patients. *Annals of Internal Medicine, 119,* 177–184.

Centers for Disease Control. (1991). Purified Protein Derivative (PPD)-tuberculin anergy and HIV infection: Guidelines for anergy testing and management of anergic persons at risk of tuberculosis. *Morbidity and Mortality Weekly Report, 40,* 27–33.

Clough, M. (1917). The cultivation of tubercle bacilli from the circulating blood in miliary tuberculosis. *American Review of Tuberculosis, 1,* 598–621.

Daley, C. L., Small, P. M., & Schecter, G. F. (1992). An outbreak of tuberculosis with accelerated progression among persons infected with the immunodeficiency virus; an analysis using restriction-fragment-length polymorphisms. *New England Journal of Medicine, 326,* 231–235.

Eisenstein, B. L. (1990). The polymerase chain reaction: A new diagnostic method of using molecular genetics for medical diagnosis. *New England Journal of Medicine, 322,* 178–183.

Greenbaum, M., Beyt, B. E., & Murray, P. R. (1980). The accuracy of diagnosing tuberculosis at a large teaching hospital. *American Review of Respiratory Disease, 121,* 477–481.

Jones, B. E., Young, S. M., Antoniskis, D., Davidson, P. T., Kramer, F., & Barnes, P. F. (1993). Relationship of the manifestations of tuberculosis to CD4 cell counts in patients with human immunodeficiency virus infection. *American Review of Respiratory Disease, 148,* 1292–1297.

Kennedy, D. J., Lewis, W. P., & Barnes, P. J. (1992). Yield of bronchoscopy for the diagnosis of tuberculosis in patients with human immunodeficiency virus infection. *Chest, 102,* 1040–1044.

Kim, T. C., Blackman, R. S., & Heatwole, A. M. (1984). Acid fast bacilli in sputum smears of patients with tuberculosis: Prevalence and significance of negative smears pretreatment and positive smears post treatment. *American Review of Respiratory Disease, 129,* 264–270.

Klein, N. C., Duncanson, F. P., Lennox, T. H., Pitta, A., Cohen, S. C., & Wormser, G. P. (1989). Use of mycobacterial smears in the diagnosis of pulmonary tuberculosis in AIDS/ARC patients. *Chest, 95,* 1190–1192.

Levy, H., Feldman, C., Sacho, H., van der Meulen, H., Kallenbach, J., & Koornhof, H. (1989). A reevaluation of sputum microscopy and culture in the diagnosis of pulmonary tuberculosis. *Chest, 95,* 1193–1197.

Middlebrook, G., Reggiardo, Z., & Tiggertt, W. D. (1977). Automatable radiometric detection of growth of *Mycobacterium tuberculosis* in selective media. *American Review of Respiratory Disease, 115,* 1066–1071.

New York City Department of Health. (1993). *Tuberculosis at a glance* (3rd ed.). New York: City of New York.

Patel, Y. R., Mehta, J. B., Harvill, L., & Gateley, K. (1993). Flexible bronchoscopy as a diagnostic tool in the evaluation of pulmonary tuberculosis in an elderly population. *Journal of the American Geriatrics Society, 41,* 629–632.

Pitchenik, A. E., Fertel, D., & Block A. B. (1988). Mycobacterial disease: Epidemiology, diagnosis, treatment and prevention. *Clinics in Chest Medicine, 9,* 425–441.

Selwyn, P. A., Hartel, D., & Lewis, V. A. (1989). A prospective study of the risk of tuberculosis among intravenous drug users with human immunodeficiency virus infection. *New England Journal of Medicine, 320,* 545–550.

Shafer, R. W., Goldberg R., Siera, M., & Glatt, A. E. (1989). Frequency of *Mycobacterium tuberculosis* bacteremia in patients with tuberculosis in an area endemic for AIDS. *American Review of Respiratory Disease, 140,* 1611–1613.

Sunderam, G., McDonald, R. J., Maniatis, T., Oleske, J., Kapila, R., & Reichman, L. B. (1986). Tuberculosis as a manifestation of the acquired immunodeficiency syndrome (AIDS). *Journal of the American Medical Association, 256,* 362–366.

Thompson, N. J., Glassroth, J. L., Snider, D. E., Jr., & Farer, L. S. (1979). The booster phenomenon in serial tuberculin skin testing. *American Review of Respiratory Disease, 119,* 587–597.

5

Treatment of Tuberculous Infection and Disease

Proving efficacy of any new treatment can be difficult when the natural history of a disease is unpredictable. Tuberculosis carried a mortality rate of 50% to 60% in the best of circumstances before the advent of effective antibiotic therapy in the late 1940s (New York City Department of Health, 1982). People had undoubtedly survived the disease throughout history without physicians' help. This fact probably resulted in the continuation of treatments of questionable benefit that may have actually harmed patients. There have also been many false starts along the way to a real cure.

When a disease carries a 100% mortality and a new treatment allows a patient to survive, it is readily apparent that the new treatment is a success. In 1933, when a young German woman dying of an overwhelming streptococcal infection complicated by renal failure was treated with Prontosil, the first sulfonamide antibiotic, her rapid and complete recovery was so dramatic that there could be no question about the efficacy of the drug (Ryan, 1993). When only half of all patients survive a disease like tuberculosis without treatment and a patient receiving a new treatment survives, it is only natural to believe that the new therapy was responsible. This can lead to acceptance of treatments that truly may not be effective. In other words, the patient may have gotten well independent of, or even in spite of, the treatment.

Today, before a treatment is considered effective, it must undergo evaluation in clinical trials. These are large studies that attempt to discover whether a new treatment results in a better outcome for a statistically significant proportion of patients than does the older treatment or no treatment at all. In these studies, a new treatment (treatment group) is compared to no treatment or a conventional treatment (control group). Statistical calculations are performed to demonstrate that differences between control and treatment groups are real and not due to random chance. These studies tend to be complicated, expensive, and are sometimes flawed, but they are necessary to prevent the adoption of ineffective therapies. This type of evaluation is necessary if the benefit is real, but subtle. Very few new treatments are as dramatic as Prontosil or penicillin. As an example, the antiretroviral agent zidovudine does not eradicate an HIV-1 infection, but studies have determined that for those with advanced stages of the disease, it can slow or temporarily halt progression of immune deficiency to full blown AIDS (Fishl et al., 1987). It took a carefully planned clinical trial to demonstrate this fact.

This chapter will review some of the earliest forms of tuberculosis treatment and the standard medical regimens of today. The older surgical techniques are still relevant. Because of the rise of multidrug-resistant tuberculosis (MDR-TB), some of the old surgical techniques are once again used as adjunct therapy in cases where the organisms are resistant to most of the first and second line drugs. In addition, many health professionals will have the opportunity to care for elderly individuals who underwent these procedures in the 1930s and 1940s. Often these procedures dramatically altered the physical exam and chest x-ray patterns of these individuals.

Modern chemotherapeutic regimens cure tuberculosis virtually 100% of the time, even in those with impaired immunity from HIV-1 infection. The major exception is MDR-TB. Resistant tuberculosis has always existed, but has now become much more common in urban areas. The relationship between HIV-1 infection and MDR-TB will be explored. We will discuss preventive or prophylactic treatment of tuberculous infection. Other important topics discussed will be treatment of children and pregnant women for tuberculous infection and disease. Because of various drug toxicities, different combinations of drugs must be used than in healthy, nonpregnant adults. Finally, and most important of all, the issue of compliance with chemotherapeutic regimens will be reviewed. Picking the safest, most effective regimen is relatively easy, compared to insuring that the patient is able to complete a full course of therapy. *Directly observed therapy* (DOT) is a proven method of tuberculosis treatment that may be the only way to overcome the current tuberculosis epidemic, and will be discussed as well.

PRE-ANTIBIOTIC THERAPIES OF ACTIVE TUBERCULOSIS

Before there was a proven cure for tuberculosis, various therapies were tried, some of which may seem to border on the bizarre today. These treatments included isolation from family and friends in tuberculosis sanitaria (especially for the wealthy) as well as drastic surgical procedures. In the sanitaria, the regimen initially consisted of strict bed rest, with gradually increased exercise, unusual (including high egg) diets, exposure to cold, clean mountain air, and, often, surgical procedures (Walsh, 1919). The poor man's cure was often sleeping on rooftops or fire escapes.

Surgical procedures consisted of various techniques with a common goal of mechanically compressing the lung to close the tuberculous cavity and put the lung in a resting state. It was known from careful study of the natural history of tuberculosis patients that the spontaneous closing of a tuberculous cavity could herald the beginning of arrested disease or even cure. Surgical procedures tried to duplicate this process in the hopes of a cure. For example, therapeutic pneumoperitoneum, or the intentional introduction of air into the abdominal cavity, was done to raise the diaphragm when the disease was in the lower lobes, again compressing the tuberculous cavity. Although the exact mechanism may not be known, collapsing a lung with cavitary TB can arrest the disease. Presumably this occurs because the oxygen concentration is decreased in the cavity. *Mycobacterium tuberculosis* bacilli grow best in an environment with a high oxygen content and are inhibited when oxygen levels fall.

The most common procedure was the creation of a collapsed lung or an intentional pneumothorax. In this procedure, air or an inert gas such as nitrogen was introduced through a needle inserted through the chest wall into the pleural cavity, causing the lung to collapse. Each lung sits in a hollow space in the chest cavity where a slight negative air pressure maintains the normal inflated state. If this slight negative pressure becomes positive, the lung will partially collapse. In the most desperate cases of MDR-TB today, this technique is still used with some benefit (Iseman & Madsen, 1989).

Perhaps the most dramatic procedure of all was the thoracoplasty, or the removal of from 2 to 9 ribs in an attempt to cure the patient of tuberculosis by decreasing the volume of the chest cavity. By the late 1930s this technique was refined to the point where 80% of those undergoing the procedure had closure of cavities and elimination of organisms from sputum smears. Although pulmonary function was distorted, patients were usually able to resume fairly normal functioning after the procedure (Ayvazian, 1993).

How did such strange procedures come about? It must be remembered that prior to the age of antibiotics in the 1930s there was no medicinal cure for any infection. Infections such as abscesses were treated surgically, while a simple cellulitis was often fatal. Prior to Robert Koch's discovery of the causative agent of tuberculosis in 1882, it wasn't clear that tuberculosis was due to a microorganism. Treatment was based on trying to duplicate spontaneous conditions which seemed to occur in patients who recovered. It was suggested as early as 1771 by Edmond Claud Bourru of the Faculté de Médecin in Paris that a pneumothorax, by helping close the pulmonary tuberculosis cavity, could be of benefit in the treatment of pulmonary tuberculosis. In the Cook County Infirmary, J. B. Murphy had noted that Civil War chest wounds resulting in pneumothoraxes did not cause serious problems by themselves. Wounded solders usually survived these episodes. The first artificial pneumothorax as a treatment of tuberculosis was induced in 1888 by Carlo Forlanini in Italy. During the next 18 years, he documented 25 cases of induced pneumothorax treatment of active tuberculosis. In this era, tuberculosis was sometimes treated as lung cancer is today, with removal of a lobe or entire lung being the only chance for cure. Today, in cases of MDR-TB, removal of infected lung tissue, along with complicated chemotherapeutic regimens, is used to treat the most difficult cases (Iseman & Madsen, 1989).

The pessimistic spirit of the times with regard to tuberculosis is hard for us to imagine. In the movie *The Bells of St. Mary's* (1945), Bing Crosby played a pastor at a small, poor parish school forced to send the principal (Ingrid Bergman) away to a sanitarium because she had a "touch" of tuberculosis. The impact lost on the audience of today is that this parish school principal had a disease with a 50% 5-year mortality rate. She was not being sent away for rest and cure, but in all probability to die. The use of streptomycin or para-aminosalicylic acid (PAS) was still years away, and routine cures still awaited the arrival of combination chemotherapy. Perhaps the current pessimism with AIDS therapies would be a valid comparison with the view of most medical personnel in 1945 regarding a real cure for tuberculosis. It took 65 years from the discovery of the etiology of tuberculosis to an effective cure. It is now only 9 years since HIV-1 was discovered, and yet pessimism abounds both within and without the medical community.

PREVENTIVE THERAPY

The majority of those infected with *Mycobacterium tuberculosis* do not develop active tuberculosis. Looking at all persons with tuberculous infection in the United States, only about 10% will develop tuberculosis during their lifetimes (Centers for Disease Control [CDC], 1991a). There are certain risk factors which make it more likely for some individuals to develop active tuberculosis. Preventive therapy, or prophylaxis, usually centers on these individuals. The goal of preventive therapy is to lessen the chances of progressing to active disease, maintain the health of the individual, and hasten the elimination of tuberculosis by preventing its spread. *Mycobacterium tuberculosis* cannot survive for long outside of its human host. If those with active tuberculosis are effectively treated, and those with tuberculous infection are given effective preventive treatment, tuberculosis, like smallpox, could be eliminated forever.

The best studied preventive treatment is the oral administration of isoniazid (INH) for periods of 6 to 12 months to those infected with *M. tuberculosis,* as indicated by positive tuberculin skin tests. It is possible, however (as discussed in chapter 4), to harbor a tuberculous infection, and, for many reasons, not give an appropriate (positive) response to PPD. Decisions about preventive therapy in this situation will be discussed later.

The efficacy of INH has been demonstrated in extensive trials by the United States Public Health Service, as well as other large studies (Ferebee, 1970). To date, long-term follow-up of individuals treated prophylactically with INH demonstrates consistent, significant (nearly tenfold) reduction in the rate of progression to active tuberculosis. This protection appears to last for 20 years or more and is presumably lifelong (American Thoracic Society, 1983).

Although all persons infected with *Mycobacterium tuberculosis* are thought to benefit from preventive treatment, there is the question of possible isoniazid toxicity to consider. Deciding whom and why to treat is based on the risk of development of active tuberculous disease versus the risk of isoniazid hepatotoxicity.

Establishing Guidelines for Preventive Treatment

In order to assess the benefits and risks of a particular preventive treatment, one must know three things: (a) the risk of developing the disease without treatment, (b) the effectiveness of the treatment in preventing the disease, and (c) the potential toxicity of the treatment. Guidelines can then be created for recommending or not recommending treatment. Treatment of tuberculous infection and disease has been available for nearly 50 years and these guidelines are well established.

Risk of Development of Active Tuberculosis

Only 10% of those with normal immunity who are infected with *Mycobacterium tuberculosis* will ever develop active disease (CDC, 1991a). Those who do develop tuberculosis do so within the first 2 years of the primary infection or, often, many years later, presumably because of other immune-compromising medical disorders and aging (CDC, 1992a). The infected state is usually demonstrated by a significant response to an intradermal injection of 5 TU of PPD-S. (Refer to chapter 4, "Diagnosis of Tuberculous Infection.") This 10% lifetime risk for development of active tuberculosis is an average, composed of thousands of individuals, a range including a white 60-year-old Iowa farmer and a 28-year-old African American resident of a shelter for homeless persons in New York. Such individuals may have very different medical problems and access to medical care. They also may have very different risks of developing active tuberculosis.

From years of study, it is possible to estimate the increased risk for development of active tuberculosis in individuals with certain health problems compared with infected persons with no known risk factor (see Table 1.2). Prior to the emergence of HIV disease, certain medical problems affecting immunity or certain life circumstances increased some individuals' risk of developing tuberculosis from 2 to 16 times. These factors ranged from the age of the person becoming infected, to the recentness of infection, to known immunocompromising conditions. The very young (≤5 years old) and the elderly (>60 years old) carry a risk of progressing from infection to disease from 2.2 to 5.0 times the risk of someone outside of these age groups. Those who have progressed from a negative tuberculin skin test to a positive one within the past 2 years (i.e., "recent converters") have a risk of development of active disease that is 15.0 times greater than those with longstanding positive tuberculin skin tests. Persons with altered immunity from non-HIV sources are also at increased risk for progression to active tuberculosis. Medical conditions such as diabetes mellitus type I, renal failure, carcinoma of the head and neck, and iatrogenic immunosuppression can increase the likelihood of progression to active tuberculosis from 3.6 to 16.0 times over that of an individual without one of these problems. Iatrogenic suppression of immunity can result from high-dose corticosteroid use (necessary treatment in various illnesses) or from cancer chemotherapy. Patients receiving such therapy often have periods of extremely low white blood cell counts while their bone marrow recovers from the effects of the treatment.

The appearance of HIV infection and its profound disturbance to cell-mediated immunity, the main line of defense against active tuberculosis, has changed the whole picture. The effects of HIV on a person's ability to prevent tuberculous infection from progressing to disease are 10 times greater than any of the immune problems discussed above. One early study looked into the risk of development of active tuberculosis in HIV-infected individuals attending a methadone maintenance program in New York City. These researchers found an annual risk of

7%, compared to a lifetime risk of 10% for developing active tuberculosis (Selwyn et al., 1989). Stated differently, the risk of development of active tuberculosis in an HIV-infected individual may be 100 to 200 times greater than the risk of tuberculosis in a non–HIV-infected individual. This brings a whole new sense of urgency to INH prophylaxis. Before HIV, physicians preventively treated patients infected with *M. tuberculosis* even though many would not have developed active tuberculosis without the treatment. Although there were certain medical conditions which increased the likelihood of developing active tuberculosis, none could compare with HIV infection as a risk factor. Now, we may need to treat all dually infected (HIV and *M. tuberculosis*) individuals preventively because every single one of them may develop active disease without treatment.

Effectiveness of Isoniazid Prophylaxis

Isoniazid prophylaxis has been described as being from 30%–93% effective in preventing the development of active tuberculosis in those infected with *M. tuberculosis,* as evidenced by a positive tuberculin skin test. This variability is probably due to differences in patient compliance with the prescribed regimen. A study of Arkansas nursing home residents (where compliance was less of an issue) demonstrated much better results. There was a 98% reduction in the rate of development of active disease in those with documented tuberculin skin test conversions who completed a 12 month regimen of isoniazid compared with those who did not take the medication (Stead, To, Harrison, & Abraham, 1987).

   What is known about the efficacy of isoniazid prophylaxis in those with HIV infection? Studies demonstrating the efficacy of INH go back several decades before the current HIV pandemic and, therefore, included comparatively immune-intact individuals. We are only now beginning to gather the same type of information for individuals coinfected with *M. tuberculosis* and HIV. An early report from a recent study in Zambia shows an 87% reduction in the rate of active disease in those tuberculin-positive, HIV-infected individuals who completed a 6-month regimen of INH compared to those who received placebo (Wadhawan, Hira, Mwansa, Tembo, & Perine, 1991). Isoniazid preventive therapy is not only effective in persons with relatively intact immunity, but probably in those infected with HIV as well.

Potential Toxicity of Isoniazid

Like all medications, isoniazid can cause side effects. Side effects can be thought of as unexpected reactions to a medication or treatment that occur in some individuals. Side effects are the exception rather than the rule with medications. An effective drug with frequent, severe side effects would never be approved for use in humans, unless the condition being treated were frequently fatal without treatment. Thus, the toxic side effects of cancer chemotherapy and antiretroviral therapies are tolerated because the conditions they treat are lifethreatening without treatment. Headache remedies, on the other hand, such as acetaminophen (Tylenol®) or aspirin, are among the safest drugs available, and are available without a prescription.

Isoniazid lies somewhere in between these two extremes. The overwhelming majority of patients can take it without any untoward effects. A minority of patients, however, will suffer toxicity, usually in the form of isoniazid hepatitis. Hepatitis literally means 'inflammation of the liver'. Although there are many causes, most cases of hepatitis are due to either infectious agents (viruses, etc.) or drugs (including alcohol). Liver function can be monitored by measurement of certain liver enzymes in the blood, called aminotransferases. Probably 10% to 20% of all persons taking INH will show slight elevation of these enzymes (such as SGOT and SGPT) reflecting some mild liver dysfunction (American Thoracic Society, 1983). Enzyme levels usually return to normal despite continuation of therapy, but in a small percentage of individuals the levels will continue to rise, indicating significant liver damage and frank hepatitis (with jaundice) can occur. Like most types of chemically induced hepatitis, this usually resolves when the offending agent (isoniazid) is discontinued. Rarely, there have been deaths reported from isoniazid hepatitis. Although the exact mechanism of isoniazid induced hepatitis is not fully known, we do know that the frequency of hepatitis increases with age (Table 5.1). Daily consumption of alcohol is also believed to increase the likelihood of developing INH hepatitis.

Peripheral neuropathy is another potential side effect of INH. Isoniazid is believed to interfere with the metabolism of pyridoxine, or vitamin B-6. This is uncommon at the dose normally used to treat pulmonary tuberculosis (5 mg/kg). When patients have medical conditions

TABLE 5.1 Incidence of Isoniazid Hepatitis Versus Age

Age in years	Incidence of INH hepatitis (%)
0–19	0.0
20–34	0.3
35–49	1.2
<50	2.3

Source: Centers for Disease Control/American Thoracic Society (1983). Treatment of tuberculosis and other mycobacterial diseases. *American Review of Respiratory Disease; 127,* 790–796.

which predispose them to peripheral neuropathies, such as uremia or diabetes mellitus, or have inadequate nutritional intake, which may be associated with homelessness, alcoholism, or drug dependency, it is recommended that oral pyridoxine supplements (25 to 50 mg) be given along with INH.

Current Recommendations for Preventive Therapy of Tuberculous Infection

By examining the risk of development of active tuberculosis from the tuberculous infected state, the effectiveness of preventive therapy, and the risk of toxicity, guidelines have been established for treatment of tuberculous infection based on tuberculin skin testing (Table 5.2). It should be noted that the definition of what constitutes a positive tuberculin skin test varies according to other associated medical problems, or the circumstances surrounding the test. For persons with known or suspected HIV infection, contacts of newly diagnosed infectious tuberculosis cases, and previously untreated persons with chest x-rays consistent with old tuberculosis, 5 mm of induration is considered a positive tuberculin skin test. Ten millimeters of induration is considered positive for recent tuberculin skin test converters, intravenous drug users (HIV negative), those with other medical conditions that increase the risk of tuberculosis, foreign-born persons from high-prevalence countries, persons from medically underserved populations, and residents of long-term-care facilities. Finally, for persons under 35 years old not belonging to any of the groups above, 15 mm is considered to be a positive tuberculin skin test.

TABLE 5.2 Guidelines for Isoniazid Preventive Therapy

Skin-test positive persons in the following high-risk groups, regardless of age:
- Persons with known or suspected HIV infection (≥5 mm)
- Close contacts of infectious tuberculosis cases (≥5 mm)
- Recent tuberculin skin test converters (≥10 mm increase within a two year period for those less than 35 years old; ≥15 mm increase for those age 35 years and older)
- Previously untreated or inadequately treated persons with abnormal chest radiographs (≥5 mm)
- Intravenous drug users (≥10 mm)
- Persons with medical conditions that increase the risk of tuberculosis (≥10 mm) (see Table 5.3)

Skin-test positive persons in the following high-risk groups who are less than 35 years of age:
- Foreign-born persons from high-prevalence countries
- Medically underserved, low-income populations, including high-risk minorities
- Residents of long-term-care facilities (including prisons, shelters, and nursing homes)

Source: Centers for Disease Control/American Thoracic Society (1991, April). *The Core Curriculum on Tuberculosis* (2nd Ed.).

The usual regimen of preventive therapy is isoniazid 300 mg per day for 6 to 12 months. Those persons with chest x-rays consistent with past (and untreated) tuberculosis and those with HIV infection should receive 12 months of treatment. Persons in the remaining categories should receive 6 months of treatment. Isoniazid can also be administered in a twice-weekly regimen at a dose of 15 mg/kg (up to 900 mg) in circumstances when it would be difficult to directly observe daily therapy and compliance is a problem. The total twice weekly dosage is less because to simply divide seven days medication into 2 (2,100 mg/2 = 1,050 mg) results in unacceptable rates of toxicity. A dose of 900 mg twice a week is safe *and* just as effective as 300 mg QD. The relapse rate is no higher with twice a week dosing. The biggest obstacle to completion of therapy is not drug toxicity, but noncompliance with medication. Patients are asked to take a medication on a daily basis for several months to a year for an asymptomatic condition. Patients on therapy for active disease experience the positive reinforcement of improvement or reversal of symptoms (fever, cough, night sweats, and weight loss). Patients on preventive therapy should feel no different while on or after therapy than they did before. If they do experience any change in the way they feel, it may signal adverse effects of the isoniazid. Furthermore, many persons with tuberculous infection are impoverished, and/or homeless and may have much more pressing needs than preventive therapy, such as the struggle to obtain food and shelter each night.

Tuberculin skin testing performed in conjunction with anergy skin testing sometimes reveals a false-negative result. The individual is incapable of mounting an appropriate cutaneous response to an intradermal injection of any antigen. Because of the enhanced risk of development of active tuberculosis in severely immunosuppressed persons with HIV, the Centers for Disease Control and American Thoracic Society recommend INH preventive therapy in certain circumstances with a negative tuberculin skin test. Preventive therapy is recommended for anergic individuals with HIV infection if the local population has a 10% or higher tuberculous infection rate (CDC, 1991b). If the prevalence of tuberculous infection in the community is 10% or greater, these patients should be offered preventive therapy.

The guidelines for preventive therapy as described assume that the person is infected with a strain of M. tuberculosis that is not resistant to isoniazid or other antituberculous drugs. In the past, multidrug-resistant tuberculosis (MDR-TB) was rare. Recently, there have been outbreaks in hospitals, residential facilities for HIV-infected persons, drug treatment programs, and prisons (CDC, 1991c, 1992b; Daley et al., 1992; Edlin et al., 1992). If an individual becomes infected with a strain of M. tuberculosis resistant only to INH, the recommended prophylactic agent is rifampin (RIF), given in a dose of 600 mg each day for 12 months (American Thoracic Society, 1986).

Confronted with the possibility that an individual has become infected with a strain of M. tuberculosis resistant to both INH and RIF, several steps must be taken to help decide the most appropriate therapy. There are three factors to consider in the approach to such an individual (CDC, 1992a): (a) the likelihood that the contact is newly infected with M. tuberculosis, (b) the likelihood that the infecting strain of M. tuberculosis is multidrug-resistant, and (c) the estimated likelihood that the contact, if infected, will develop active tuberculosis.

The determination that a person is newly infected with M. tuberculosis is done by serial tuberculin skin testing. Knowing the circumstances under which the person became infected will help decide if it was likely to have been with a multidrug-resistant strain. Factors such as the degree of infectiousness of the source case, the closeness and intensity of the exposure, and the contact's risk of exposure to drug-susceptible tuberculosis will help decide the likelihood of infection with MDR-TB. A careful medical history and physical exam with special attention to immune-related disorders (HIV, etc.) will help predict the likelihood of the infected individual developing active tuberculosis. Those who appear to have been recently infected with a multidrug-resistant (MDR) strain of *M. tuberculosis,* and especially those contacts who appear to be at enhanced risk for developing active tuberculosis, should be offered multidrug preventive therapy.

Although INH is currently the only drug approved by the Food and Drug Administration (FDA) as a prophylactic agent, CDC does make several recommendations concerning possible choices of alternative therapy (CDC, 1992a):

1. Pyrazinamide (PZA), daily oral dose 25–30 mg/kg, and etham-butol (EMB), daily oral dose 15–25 mg/kg, may be given for 6 to 12 months.
2. PZA and a fluoroquinolone are suggested, although long-term study of fluoroquinolones has not been done.
3. Aminoglycosides could be considered for alternative therapy, although they must be given by daily injection, and have oto- and nephrotoxicity.
4. Para-aminosalicylic acid (PAS), ethionamide, and cycloserine are not recommended for alternative preventive therapy because of their limited efficacy and high frequency of side effects.

TREATMENT OF ACTIVE TUBERCULOSIS

Treatment of active tuberculosis is based on two important bacteriolog-ical principles (American Thoracic Society, 1983): (a) the existence of spontaneous mutant organisms resistant to a single antituberculous medication, and (b) the persistence of viable mycobacteria, due to their slow or intermittent growth.

Because of these two principles, treatment of active tuberculosis dis-ease consists of multiple drugs taken together consistently for 6 to 18 months or longer. The odds of a single organism being resistant to an antituberculous drug (possessing "native resistance") without prior exposure is about one in a million (1×10^6). The average cavitary lesion in tuberculosis contains about a billion (1×10^9) organisms, meaning there are probably 1,000 (1×10^3) organisms already resistant to a single antituberculous agent. If only a single drug were used, there would be an initial favorable response as the overwhelming number of susceptible organisms die. Then there would be selective growth of resistant organisms, and soon the entire population of organisms in that patient would be resistant to that single drug. The patient would improve initially and then steadily deteriorate and perhaps die. This is exactly what happened when streptomycin, and then para-aminosalicylic acid (PAS), the first effective antituberculous drugs, were used alone. Although there were many apparent cures, the majority of patients (especially with streptomycin) experienced relapses within the next several years (Ryan, 1993). It was not until drugs were used in combination that the first reliable cures were obtained. The odds of a single organism being resistant to two drugs it has never seen before would be the product of each individual probability:

$$1 \times 10^{-6} \times 1 \times 10^{-6} = 1 \times 10^{-12}$$

It would take 1,000 patients with cavitary lesions to find a single organism resistant to both drugs. Unfortunately, active disease caused by susceptible organisms can develop drug resistance through inadequate dosing. Multiple starts and stops in therapy also allow drug-resistant organisms to flourish. This secondary drug resistance can develop in a matter of months. It was first seen in the initial monotherapy of active tuberculosis with streptomycin in the 1940s which resulted in 90% of patients having drug-resistant organisms in sputum specimens after 4 months of therapy (Ryan, 1993). In addition, individuals can develop active tuberculosis from an initial infection with MDR organisms. This is called primary drug resistance. In recent years, multidrug-resistant tuberculosis (MDR-TB) has gone from being an aberration occurring in a few isolated cases to being a commonplace occurrence in major urban centers.

The second bacteriologic consideration is the persistence of *M. tuberculosis* organisms because of slow or intermittent growth. Persons can become ill with active tuberculosis decades after their initial infection. *Mycobacterium tuberculosis* can grow very slowly or remain dormant for several decades. There are believed to be three populations of organisms that can be treated with antituberculous drugs. The largest population exists extracellularly and is actively growing. It is from this population that drug resistance arises. Another smaller group survives within the acidic environment of macrophages and grows slowly or intermittently. The third group exists in the neutral pH of caseous granulomas, and also grows very slowly or intermittently. The various antituberculous drugs work best in different populations and environments.

Antibiotics for tuberculosis are usually either bacteriostatic or bactericidal against *M. tuberculosis*. A bacteriostatic drug halts cellular reproduction, but when the drug is withdrawn, the organism is free to return to its former active metabolic state. Bacteriostatic drugs can be used in combination therapy, but today would never be used alone for either preventive therapy or treatment of active disease. As the name implies, bactericidal drugs actually can kill *Mycobacterium tuberculosis*. Rifampin is bactericidal in all three environments among all three populations. Isoniazid is bactericidal against dividing organisms in cavitary lesions as well as those in macrophages. The aminoglycosides like streptomycin are bactericidal only against actively dividing extracellular organisms. Pyrazinamide is bactericidal only for intracellular organisms. All of the remaining antituberculous drugs are only bacteriostatic.

Treatment Regimens for Drug-Sensitive Organisms

Pulmonary Tuberculosis

Regimens for treatment of active tuberculosis vary little between those who are co-infected with HIV and those who are not. The main difference is in the duration of treatment. In an ideal world, a newly diagnosed, never previously treated case of tuberculosis can be cured in 6 months, assuming the person's immune system is intact. This also assumes that the person's disease is not from an organism resistant to two or more drugs (multidrug-resistant). Often even these uncomplicated patients end up receiving longer treatment, usually because of lapses in therapy.

The treatment of active tuberculosis is chronic and cumulative. Each day's therapy adds to the previous day's to provide a continuous hostile environment to *M. tuberculosis.* Lapses in therapy encourage the growth of those organisms most resistant to the drugs being used. After repeated lapses, the population of unkilled, resistant organisms is free to grow logarithmically.

To minimize the risk of development of MDR-TB, and to ensure that the patient gets at least two effective drugs, new guidelines have been established describing initial therapy of new cases of tuberculosis. Since December, 1991, in New York City, initial therapy of new, previously untreated tuberculosis consists of four antituberculous medications (New York City Department of Health, 1992):

- Isoniazid (INH) 300 mg per day
- Rifampin (RIF) 600 mg per day
- Pyrazinamide (PZA) 20 to 30 mg/kg per day
- Ethambutol (EMB) 15 to 25 mg/kg per day

Recently, the American Thoracic Society and the Centers for Disease Control and Prevention issued updated guidelines for initial treatment regimens (American Thoracic Society & Centers for Disease Control and Prevention,1994). They offer 3 options:

- INH, RIF, and PZA for 8 weeks, then INH and RIF for 16 weeks (If local INH resistance rates are >4%, ETH should be added for the first 8 weeks.)
- Daily INH, RIF, PZA, and streptomycin or ETH for 2 weeks, then all 4 drugs twice weekly for 6 weeks by directly observed therapy (DOT). At the 7th week, PZA and streptomycin or ETH are dropped and INH and RIF are continued twice weekly for 16 weeks by DOT.
- INH, RIF, PZA, and streptomycin or ETH 3 times weekly by DOT for 6 months.

All three regimens carry a specific warning to consult a tuberculosis medical expert if the patient remains symptomatic or smear- or culture-positive after 3 months. The advantage to using 3 or 4 drugs is that the duration of therapy can be reduced to as little as 6 months with approximately the same cure rate, improved compliance, and no greater toxicity than when 2 drugs are used (Combs, O'Brien, & Geiter, 1990).

Because of the rise of MDR-TB, patients need to be treated initially with 4 drugs. If the patient's illness has underlying resistance to INH and RIF, he or she will still be on 2 other effective drugs while waiting for exhibition of drug sensitivities. Although there are faster turn-around times at specialized centers for tuberculosis treatment, most labs require about 6 to 8 weeks for drug sensitivities. If the initial culture results show no drug resistance patterns, the PZA and EMB are usually dropped and INH and RIF are continued for another 6 months. The need to adjust the regimen after sensitivities are known explains the need for using so many drugs in the initial phase of tuberculosis therapy.

Those tuberculosis patients coinfected with HIV are usually treated longer than those not coinfected (Figure 5.1). The minimum course of treatment is 9 months for organisms that are sensitive to the usual drugs. It appears that present antituberculous regimens work well in HIV-infected individuals, if there is no drug resistance (Small et al., 1991).

Extrapulmonary Tuberculosis

The regimens for extrapulmonary tuberculosis are basically the same as for pulmonary tuberculosis. Although controlled clinical trials for optimum treatment regimens in extrapulmonary tuberculosis have not been conducted to the same extent as with pulmonary tuberculosis, the standard regimens appear to be effective and are usually recommended (Dutt & Stead, 1989).

Treatment Regimens for Drug-Resistant Organisms

Drug resistance, especially multidrug resistance, has become an increasing problem in tuberculosis treatment. When a strain of *Myco-bacterium tuberculosis* is resistant to an antibiotic, that drug is unable to kill or arrest the reproduction of the organism at the usual doses. As mentioned earlier, naturally occurring wild mutant bacilli can be resis-

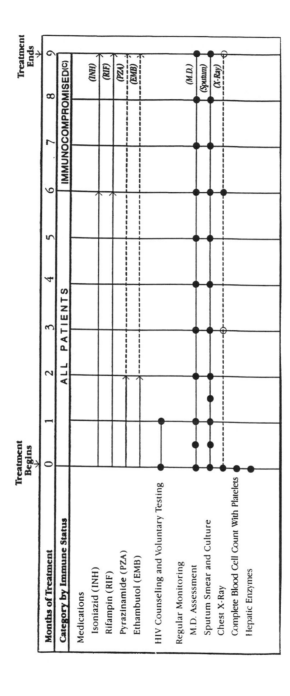

FIGURE 5.1　Therapy timeline for previously untreated tuberculosis patients with active disease. *Source:* New York City Department of Health (1992). Tuberculosis Treatment. *City Health Information, 11*(5), 1–4. (Available from City Health Information, 125 Worth Street, Rm. 326, Box 77, New York, NY 10013).

tant to an antibiotic they have never seen. This is why two drugs are needed to cure tuberculosis. The odds of having even a single organism naturally resistant to both antituberculous drugs is probably 1,000 times greater than the number of organisms in the patient. Because of this, as recently as 1985, the standard initial treatment for uncomplicated pulmonary tuberculosis was either 2 or 3 drugs. Most often used was isoniazid and rifampin for 9 months, sometimes supplemented in the initial phase of 2 to 8 weeks with ethambutol, streptomycin, or pyrazinamide.

Single drug or multidrug resistance existed before HIV was discovered. In New York City, the percent of isolates resistant to one or more antituberculous drugs increased from 10% in 1982–1983 to 23% in 1991. During the same period, those isolates resistant to both isoniazid and rifampin increased from 3% to 7% (Frieden et al., 1993).

A recent study in New York looked at all specimens collected there in the month of April, 1991. They found that for that month, 19% of all isolates from 466 patients were resistant to both isoniazid and rifampin. Broken down further, 30% of those with a prior history of antituberculous treatment showed this multidrug-resistant (MDR) pattern, compared to only 9% of those without a history of prior treatment (Frieden et al., 1993).

In the preceding section, rates of drug resistance were given, with spontaneous, wild mutants occurring on the order of 1 in 10^6 or 0.0001% of organisms. If this were the only source of drug resistance, it would be a rare event. Unfortunately, with power to cure tuberculosis comes the ability to transform a strain into a multidrug-resistant strain. Repeatedly stopping and restarting drug regimens has the effect of selecting out those organisms which are resistant to one or more drugs and allowing them to multiply unimpeded, resulting in acquired, or secondary drug resistance. A person who is initially infected and develops disease from a drug resistant organism experiences *primary drug resistance*. The study from New York cited earlier demonstrated primary drug resistance to isoniazid and rifampin in 7% of those of persons with isolates from April, 1991 (Frieden et al., 1993). These unfortunate individuals can develop active tuberculosis that carries a cure rate of 50% to 60%, compared to essentially a 100% cure rate for sensitive organisms (Iseman & Madsen, 1989; Goble et al., 1993). In the New York study, 125 of 466 patients (27%) died during the follow-up period. The most important predictors of mortality were the presence of AIDS, increasing age, and the presence of drug resistance. The overall case fatality rate was 91% for those patients with both AIDS and MDR-TB (Frieden et al., 1993). The management of patients with established MDR-TB should be left to qualified, experienced specialists in pulmonary medicine or infectious disease. It is beyond the scope of this book to cover this type of information in great detail. Each management plan is highly individualized, but there are general principles for the primary care provider which can help prevent many new cases of MDR-TB.

1. Always begin treatment of new (i.e., previously untreated) tuberculosis cases with 4 drugs while waiting for drug sensitivities (unless INH drug resistance is known to be <4% in the community).
2. When sensitivities are known, and drug resistance is not present (after about 2 months), discontinue EMB and PZA and continue INH and RIF at least another 4 months.
3. If drug resistance is suspected because of a history of prior treatment or failure to respond to treatment, *never* add just a single antituberculous agent to the standard regimen. If drug resistance is present, adding a single agent may promote further drug resistance to the single new drug. Always add at least two or more new drugs after consultation with someone experienced in this area.
4. Give the patient every chance to complete the full course of therapy. Seriously consider enrolling every new tuberculosis patient in a directly observed therapy (DOT) program.

Surgical Treatment of Pulmonary Tuberculosis

As discussed earlier, before effective antituberculous chemotherapy was developed, surgical procedures such as creation of an intentional pneumothorax, pneumoperitoneum, and even thoracoplasty were performed in an attempt to close the cavitary lesion in patients with pulmonary tuberculosis. Today there is still a place for surgical procedures in the most desperate cases where conventional treatment has failed. Several indications for surgical treatment of pulmonary tuberculosis were recommended by McLaughlin and Hankins in 1974.

- Active localized disease not responding to chemotherapy, including infection with atypical bacteria
- Residual foci of disease in patients in whom social or medical indications of potential reactivation exist or foci which interfere with proper pulmonary function or toilet function
- The possibility of coexisting carcinoma
- Various complications of pulmonary and pleural tuberculosis, including empyema, bronchopleural fistula, and massive hemorrhage from a cavitary lesion
- Management of complications following resection for tuberculosis

A more recent list of indications for surgical intervention in pulmonary tuberculosis would exclude resection of residual foci following completion of chemotherapy, since it is clear that these areas are not a source of recurrent disease once the patient has completed a full course of therapy with effective medications. This updated list of indications for surgery includes (Harris, 1994)

- Life-threatening hemoptysis
- Bronchopleural fistula formation secondary to tuberculosis
- Bronchial stenosis, as demonstrated by an opaque, airless lung on chest x-ray
- Loculated tuberculous empyema requiring pleural decortication

Surgery would be contraindicated for treatment of drug-resistant tuberculosis if the risk of surgery were high because of other medical problems. Perioperative mortality should be <1%. The patient's pulmonary reserve must be adequate to compensate for the loss of the lung tissue. Objective measurements of lung function include post-exercise arterial blood gases and ventilation-perfusion (V/Q) scanning. A patient should be able to demonstrate the ability to oxygenate adequately after mild exercise, such as walking down a flight of stairs. If a patient cannot do this, postoperative weaning from the respirator may be difficult.

A ventilation-perfusion scan measures the fraction of total ventilation performed by each lung. The two measurements are usually not equal. If the lung most affected by MDR-TB were providing a small fraction of the total ventilation, surgical resection of the affected area or the entire lung might be possible without severe pulmonary compromise.

If the contralateral lung is also heavily affected by tuberculosis, then surgery may not be the answer. If there is active endobronchial tuberculosis in the area to be resected (as confirmed by bronchoscopy), surgery must be delayed until it resolves. Usually, the medical regimen is maximized prior to surgery for the most medical benefit. If the organisms are susceptible only to two bacteriostatic drugs, then surgery should probably be earlier rather than later.

Risks of Surgery

As mentioned above, surgical risk should be <1%. Complications can include deterioration and failure of the bronchial stump (bronchial stump "blowout"). If the contents of the lung being removed spill into the pleural space, a tuberculous empyema can result. The contents of the resected lung may spill into the remaining lung, resulting in bronchogenic spread. Despite these risks, being HIV-infected is not by itself be a contraindication to surgical treatment. On the other hand, if the patient has advanced HIV disease, he or she may be so debilitated that they would be at high risk for perioperative complications and surgery cannot be done.

TREATMENT OF TUBERCULOSIS
IN PREGNANCY

To treat women with tuberculosis during pregnancy, care must be taken to choose a regimen which is both effective and safe for the woman and the fetus. In the past, drugs would be routinely administered to women without much thought to potential teratogenicity. After fetal malformations occurred with thalidomide in the late 1950s, it was apparent just how dangerous medications can be for a developing fetus. Standard medical practice now is to avoid all drugs in pregnant women unless absolutely necessary.

Preventive Therapy in Pregnancy

A pregnant woman with a positive tuberculin skin test should have a chest x-ray (with proper abdominal shielding) after the 12th week of gestation to rule out active tuberculosis (Vallejo & Starke, 1992). If the chest x-ray, history, physical exam, and specimens for AFB smear and culture are all negative for active disease, preventive treatment is usually offered in the postpartum period. A woman with a documented and recent tuberculous infection or co-infected with HIV-1 should be offered preventive therapy because of the high risk of development of active disease (CDC, 1992a). Very little antituberculous medication finds its way into breast milk, and breastfeeding should not be discouraged for fear of toxicity to the newborn. Insufficient amounts of antituberculous drugs find their way into breast milk to provide adequate therapy for tuberculous infection or active disease (O'Brien, 1993).

Treatment of Active Tuberculosis in Pregnancy

The discovery of active tuberculosis in a pregnant woman calls for immediate treatment as in any nonpregnant patient, although special considerations must be taken into account when planning a regimen. Of the first line antituberculous drugs, a regimen of isoniazid (INH), rifampin (RIF), and ethambutol (EMB) is the recommended initial treatment of tuberculosis in pregnancy (Snider, Layde, Hohnson, & Lyle, 1980). Streptomycin and other aminoglycosides can cause ototoxicity in the fetus and consequent permanent hearing loss in the child. Pyrazinamide is not recommended as an antituberculous agent in the United States because very little is known about its effects on the fetus. It is a relatively new drug, and although it has not been associated with teratogenic effects, PZA is not recommended for use in pregnancy in this country (American Thoracic Society & Centers for Disease Control and Prevention, 1994). The World Health Organization and International Union Against Tuberculosis and Lung Disease do recommend its use in the initial treatment of pregnant women (O'Brien, 1993). The length of the course of treatment would be the same as in the nonpregnant patient.

TREATMENT OF TUBERCULOSIS
IN CHILDREN

Preventive Therapy

Preventive therapy with isoniazid should be administered to children as per the guidelines mentioned earlier in this chapter for adults. Doses should be adjusted for weight. In the child with concomitant HIV infection, prophylactic treatment with isoniazid should be given for a period of 12 months, as with adults. If the child (regardless of immune status) is believed infected with organisms that are isoniazid resistant, then another drug, such as rifampin, should be used for 12 months (CDC, 1991a). In the case of exposure to multidrug resistant tuberculosis, the treatment plan needs to be tailored to the sensitivity pattern of the index case. This should be done with the advice of an expert in this field.

Because of the risk of development of active tuberculosis in the child infected through, or even exposed to, a household contact, treatment is usually initiated regardless of the initial PPD result. There are two reasons for this. Even in the child with an intact immune system, it can take 2 to 10 weeks after exposure for a positive PPD to develop. Second, in the case of a child with impaired immunity, he or she may never develop an appropriate positive tuberculin skin test result. In addition, as we have seen in Table 1.2, the person co-infected with HIV and *M. tuberculosis* is prone to develop active tuberculosis. It would make no sense to take a chance by waiting 3 months to repeat the PPD skin test and not treat the patient. Isoniazid toxicity is very rare in children.

Treatment of Active
Tuberculosis in Children

The treatment of tuberculosis in children has a certain urgency because of the rapid progression of disease, compared to adults. As discussed in chapter 3, tuberculosis in children most often presents as primary disease, that is, there is an immediate progression from infection to active disease. In relatively immature immune systems, hematogenous spread of the tubercle bacilli to various parts of the body occurs more commonly than in adults. Symptoms and physical findings in a young child may be more subtle and nonspecific than in an adult. This too points to the need for early appropriate treatment.

Several guiding principles have helped to define the current treatment regimens for children with tuberculosis (Starke, 1993):

1. Children tend to develop active tuberculosis as an immediate manifestation of tuberculous infection.
2. Children have an increased incidence of extrapulmonary tuberculosis compared to adults.
3. Pharmacokinetics of antituberculous drugs differ in children and adults.
4. Because of the difficulty children may have in taking medications essentially prepared for adults, it cannot be assumed that the drugs will be absorbed as in adults.

The mainstays of antituberculous drug treatment in adults, isoniazid and rifampin, are well tolerated in children. Other drugs have not been widely used, but are believed to be relatively safe when used to treat children. Ethambutol, whose major toxicity is optic neuritis, is usually reserved for suspected drug-resistant tuberculosis. Unless the practitioner is confident that the child is old enough to perform reliable color vision testing (necessary to detect early optic neuritis) ethambutol should be avoided as a first-line drug. In general, there is no evidence of increased toxicity of any of the antituberculous drugs in children compared to adults. In children less than 6 years old, pyrazinamide or streptomycin may be alternative third agents to use (CDC, 1991a).

The regimens of duration and monitoring should be the same for children as for adults (Figure 5.1). Children should be treated for 6 months with at least 3 drugs (isoniazid, rifampin, and pyrazinamide or streptomycin) unless local drug resistance rates are extremely low (Starke, 1993). An additional point to remember in treating suspected tuberculosis is that in infants, disease tends to disseminate and treatment should be early and aggressive. In children it is often difficult to obtain culture confirmation of disease, but sensitivities of the adult index case should be used to direct the specific agents used.

When HIV disease and tuberculosis coexist in children (since no substantial studies have been done), it has been recommended to treat using regimens established for adults (Barnes, Bloch, Davidson, & Snider, 1991).

MONITORING ANTITUBERCULOUS THERAPY

Because of the need to treat patients for long periods (6 to 12 months), there are ample opportunities for mishaps caused by either the doctors or the patients. A side effect of the "mainstreaming" of tuberculosis care is that many primary health care providers without the extensive experience of a specialist will manage tuberculosis patients. Prescriptions may be written for monthly supplies with refills, inviting patients to miss monthly follow-up appointments and risk undiscovered drug toxicity. Dosing may be inadequate, especially in the case of those drugs dispensed according to the patient's weight such as EMB and PZA.

Realizing these problems, several agencies have issued guidelines for the proper diagnosis and treatment of tuberculous infection and disease, including appropriate follow-up.

The American Thoracic Society (ATS) and Centers for Disease Control have periodically published statements describing current diagnostic standards as well as treatment modalities and tuberculosis control issues in various populations. In view of the current epidemic, the CDC recently published a concise booklet (1991a) entitled *Core Curriculum on Tuberculosis*. The New York City Department of Health, Bureau of Tuberculosis Control also published a summary of treatment of active tuberculosis in both normal and immune-deficient hosts. Both are available from the addresses listed with the references for this chapter.

Treatment of active tuberculosis should consist of *at least monthly* visits for uncomplicated cases. Patients should only be given prescriptions for a one month supply without refills. There are several reasons for this. In order to detect toxicity as early as possible, patients should be questioned for symptoms of drug toxicity at least monthly. The initial therapy of active tuberculosis consists of 4 drugs, three of which (INH, RIF, PZA) are hepatotoxic, and one which of (EMB) at initial doses can result in optic neuritis presenting as loss of color vision. These problems are usually reversible if detected early by discontinuing the offending medications and substituting others. If a patient develops slowly progressive symptoms of toxicity, and has no follow-up appointments for

2 or 3 months, he or she might continue the medicines and get sicker, or stop the medicines and develop active tuberculosis again. In the worst-case scenario, a patient might stop some of the medications and develop tuberculosis resistant to the other medicines, turning a curable case of tuberculosis into an incurable one.

To prevent this from happening, the factors outlined in Table 5.3 should be assessed and the steps described below should be taken at each visit in this simplified regimen.

Monthly Visits

History

1. *Review tuberculosis symptoms with patient.* There should be some improvement by the time of this first visit (loss of fever, weight gain, etc.). If there is no improvement or if there is actual worsening of

TABLE 5.3 Factors Affecting Compliance

Features of the Health Care System
- Referral process
- Clinical setting
- Demographic features of the provider

Features of the Regimen
- Duration of treatment
- Number of medications prescribed
- Frequency of dosing
- Prescription labeling
- Side effects
- Cost
- Safety lock containers
- Parenteral medications

Features of the Patient
- Lifestyle
- Social support
- Locus of control
- Demographic features of the patient
- Degree of disability
- Health beliefs

Features of the Patient–Health Care Provider Relationship

Source: Centers for Disease Control (1989). *Improving Patient Compliance in Tuberculosis Treatment Programs.* (Available from Information Services, National Center for Prevention Services, Centers for Disease Control and Prevention, 1600 Clifton Road NE, Mailstop E-08, Atlanta, GA 30333.)

symptoms, consider patient noncompliance to the medical regimen or drug resistance as a possibility.

2. *Review symptoms of drug toxicity.* This can be a good time to review symptoms of toxicity with the patient.

3. *Review compliance with therapy.* This is probably the most important area of medical history to review. If the status of compliance to the prescribed medical regimen is unknown, it can be impossible to estimate the success of the regimen. Patients can always spontaneously go into remission even while off therapy, and a careless medical practitioner may miss this possibility. By missing the lapse in treatment, the practitioner will reinforce any doubts about the need for further treatment held by the patient. The patient may temporarily improve, but has a very high risk of recurrence, compared to the patient who completes a full course of treatment.

Physical Examination

1. *Vital signs.* Temperature and weight are essential, and one would expect to see stability if not improvement in both.

2. *Chest exam.* Results of current exam should be compared to initial hospitalization exam. Ideally, the examining physician should be the same throughout. When this is not possible, meticulous record-keeping becomes important. Familiarity with a patient's presenting condition and pertinent physical findings can save the need for expensive, repetitive testing later.

3. *Abdominal exam.* Special attention should be paid to liver size, as hepatomegaly (liver enlargement) may indicate early drug toxicity.

4. *Extremities.* Look for any signs of acute arthritis, since PZA can raise uric acid levels and precipitate gout. This occurs in those with or without a prior history of gout.

5. *Neurological exam.* Attention should be paid to evaluation of peripheral nerves, for evidence of peripheral neuropathy. Isoniazid can cause a peripheral neuropathy through interference with pyridoxine (vitamin B-6) metabolism. Peripheral neuropathies usually present as a gradual loss of certain types of sensation, most marked in the lower extremities. Loss of vibratory sense is the first modality of sensation to be lost in the natural history of a peripheral neuropathy. This can be detected through the use of a simple tuning fork. The vibrating tuning

fork is held against a bony surface such as the medial or lateral malleolus of an ankle. While still vibrating, it is then placed more proximally on another bony surface such as the tibial tuberosity below the patella. The patient should feel very little or no decrease in the intensity of the vibration between the two sites. If there is a reproducible drop-off in vibratory sensation as one moves proximally, there may be an early peripheral neuropathy present.

Laboratory Examination

1. *Microscopic sputum exam.* This simple exam is one of the best measurements of continuing success of the current medical regimen. Serial monthly negative sputum smears and cultures are ongoing evidence that the organisms are sensitive to the drugs being used and indirect evidence that the patient is compliant with the medical regimen.

2. *Chest x-ray.* After an initial film as a baseline, the chest x-ray need not be repeated until therapy is completed, unless a problem develops. The chest x-ray is of limited usefulness in monitoring the progress of treatment because it lags several weeks behind the clinical state of the patient. A chest x-ray performed on a particular day demonstrates the appearance of disease as it was 4 to 6 weeks ago.

3. *Bloodwork/urine examination.* In an otherwise healthy adult under 35 years of age there is no need for routine bloodwork or urine exam unless drug toxicity is suspected. During the course of treatment a complete blood count (CBC) should be checked to ensure that the anemia usually noted at the time of the tuberculosis diagnosis is resolving. A liver panel should be obtained if any symptoms suggestive of hepatitis develop, but probably doesn't need to be checked again unless the patient has a history of liver disease or is over 35 years old. In such cases, the liver panel should be checked monthly as a routine or any time hepatotoxicity is suspected. Hepatotoxicity is a common side effect of INH, RIF, and PZA. Pyrazinamide can increase uric acid levels, which can be lowered with low-dose aspirin. If a patient develops signs or symptoms of gout, checking uric acid level can confirm the diagnosis. Evaluating urine specimens can help determine compliance and detect early renal toxicity (a possible side effect of rifampin). A mere visual exam of urine can detect the presence of rifampin by its characteristic orange color. A quick and inexpensive examination of urine

with reagent-coated strips (urine dip sticks) can detect early renal toxicity (rifampin) by the presence of protein, leukocytes, and/or erythrocytes, indicating the need for a more detailed microscopic exam.

Compliance

Patient compliance with prescribed antituberculous regimens has become a major issue. In recent years, about 75% of tuberculosis patients in the United States have been able to complete their course of treatment in 12 months. The normal short course treatment is only 6 months. Repeatedly failing to complete a course of tuberculosis treatment is believed to be the main cause of drug-resistant tuberculosis. Many are taking a fresh look at compliance or adherence to medical regimens in general.

The good news is that even in New York City, where 61% of all MDR-TB in the United States was found in 1992, the majority of tuberculosis cases (80%) are still sensitive to isoniazid and rifampin (Navarro, 1994). These cases are virtually 100% curable if the standard regimens are used correctly. It becomes the responsibility of the health care providers as well as the patient to see the course of treatment through to completion.

As in other large cities, the burden of tuberculosis in New York falls heavily on the disadvantaged. In 1991, the Central Harlem Health District had a case rate of active tuberculosis 5 times that of the city as a whole, and the city, in turn, had a case rate 5 times that of the United States as a whole. The homeless population in New York may have an active tuberculosis case rate of 750 per 100,000 persons or 75 times the national case rate.

The bulk of treatment of tuberculosis falls on the already overburdened, poorly funded public health system. Health care in this system has traditionally been provided by well-meaning but inexperienced house officers. Medication refills often take place in emergency rooms, where it can take hours to retrieve patients' charts and review the appropriateness of medical regimens. Patients willing to endure long waits in crowded clinic waiting rooms may never see the same health care provider twice. These circumstances provide many opportunities for errors to creep in. A remarkable paper in 1991 reported that 89%

of a series of tuberculosis patients discharged from a municipal hospital failed to complete a full course of therapy in the hospital clinic (Brudney & Dobkin, 1991). The major risk factors associated with becoming lost to follow-up were homelessness, alcohol or drug dependence, and the lack of an AIDS diagnosis. Those with an AIDS diagnosis were more likely to complete treatment of active tuberculosis than those without AIDS.

The development of multidrug resistance is often blamed on patient noncompliance, branding the patient as the villain. Failure on the part of clinicians to adhere to recognized guidelines for tuberculosis treatment may be another cause, according to one study (Mahmoudi & Iseman, 1993). This study examined a case series of patients with multidrug-resistant pulmonary tuberculosis referred to the National Jewish Center for Immunology and Respiratory Medicine between 1989 through 1990. They reviewed the records of each patient to determine if nonadherence to American Thoracic Society (ATS), Centers for Disease Control (CDC), or American College of Chest Physicians (ACCP) guidelines was significantly associated with the development of acquired drug resistance. Following this protocol, they discovered "errors" in management decisions in 80% (28/35) for these patients, resulting in treatment failure and acquired drug resistance. The most common errors were (a) addition of a single drug to a failing regimen, (b) failure to identify preexisting or acquired drug resistance, (c) initiation of an inadequate primary regimen, (d) failure to identify and address noncompliance, and (e) inappropriate isoniazid preventive therapy.

The cost of this specialized, intensive care including more toxic drugs and major surgery averaged about $180,000 per patient. The authors called for several important measures to help prevent future, costly mistakes and improve the quality of tuberculosis patient care. The practice of "mainstreaming" tuberculosis care may need to be reexamined. The recommendations included (a) aggressive professional education, (b) tighter control on the provisions of care for tuberculosis patients, and (c) commitment of additional resources to tuberculosis control programs.

There is a body of literature examining the problem of patient noncompliance or nonadherence to medical regimens. Some of the work is specific to tuberculosis treatment, and some is more generalized. Specific information regarding tuberculosis has been summarized by the

CDC in a booklet entitled *Improving Patient Compliance in Tuberculosis Treatment Programs* (CDC, 1989, p. 3). They define compliance as "the extent to which a person's health-related behavior, i.e. taking medication and keeping appointments, coincides with medical advice." Several factors are reviewed which are known to affect compliance (see Table 5.3).

Features of the health care system which can affect compliance include the referral process, the clinical setting, and the demographic features of the provider. Referrals should be made as soon as possible, since the longer patients must wait for an appointment, the less likelihood that they will keep the appointment. The clinic setting should be clean, easily accessible, operate during hours for the patient's convenience, and waiting times should be kept to a minimum. Patients (like most of us) will respond positively when treated with respect. The patient's time is as important as that of the clinic staff, including the physician. Studies have shown that patients forced to endure long waiting times for a visit have a greater "no show" rate that those seen promptly.

The demographic features of the provider can have a significant impact on compliance. Marketing research has shown that most people feel more comfortable with someone of their own socioeconomic status, ethnicity, or sex. Most of those with tuberculosis in the United States happen to be nonwhite men. The medical profession in the United States is still largely composed of white English-speaking males, although this is changing. Present medical school applicants are now more representative of the general population. For now, however, health care providers need to keep in mind that they may have to work hard at gaining the respect and confidence of many patients. It should not be assumed that a title and a white coat will inspire automatic compliance with a medical regimen in every patient.

Features of the regimen which can affect compliance include the duration of treatment, the number of medications taken, the frequency of dosing, prescription labeling, side effects, cost, whether safety-lock containers and parenteral (injected) medications are used. The longer the regimen, the greater the risk of noncompliance to that regimen. Tuberculosis treatment courses have decreased from 18 to 24 months in the 1950s to 6 to 12 months today. The standard initial regimen for uncomplicated tuberculosis today can consist of 11 pills or capsules to be taken once each day for an 80 kg man (one INH tablet, two RIF capsules, three EMB tablets, three PZA tablets, one vitamin B-6 tablet). A possible answer to this problem is the use of Rifater®, which is a combination of isoniazid, rifampin, and pyrazinamide in a single tablet. It has been approved by the FDA. Already available is Rifamate®, a combination capsule of isoniazid and rifampin.

Although it has not been demonstrated in controlled studies, most clinicians would agree that it is easiest for patients to take drugs only once a day and the pharmacokinetics of these drugs make this feasible and desirable. Antituberculous medications are usually prescribed in this way. A way to decrease frequency of dosing further is to prescribe medications to be taken twice weekly. This would usually not be done until after an induction period of about 2 months. Dosages have to be adjusted, and patients should be monitored closely for compliance since now 2 to 4 missed doses represent 1 to 2 weeks without therapy.

Prescriptions should be written with clear directions in a language the patient can understand. It is up to the health care provider to be sure that the patient is literate. Many patients may be embarrassed to admit they cannot read, and won't offer that information at all unless asked in a caring, nonjudgmental way.

Before beginning the regimen, patients should be warned about potential side effects. One drug in particular, rifampin, is associated with side effects that, while not life-threatening, are a source of great anxiety to patients. Rifampin is a rust-colored powder that distributes well throughout body fluids and colors them all orange, that is, tears, saliva, urine, and sweat. Contact lenses, and patients' underwear may be stained orange. Patients need to be warned about this, or they may decide to stop the rifampin on their own. Rifampin also increases metabolism of methadone, causing those on methadone maintenance to experience variable degrees of withdrawal. The patient as well as his or her methadone clinic should be consulted before starting this drug. Usually, by increasing the methadone dose in 10-mg increments, the rifampin effect can be overcome.

If patients cannot afford the medications prescribed for any illness they will not be able to comply with that regimen. Most health departments provide antituberculous medications for free, but if this is not the case, it is up to the health care providers to find a way of obtaining the medicine.

Safety-lock ("childproof") containers can create a real barrier to compliance, especially for those with arthritis or other disabilities. If there are no children in the house, then physicians can request on prescriptions that regular pill containers be used.

Some patients believe that injected medications are more potent than mere pills and would be more compliant with such a regimen. Others may dislike injections and may drop out of treatment.

There are features of the individual patient which may affect compliance. A patient's life situation can be a determinant of compliance. Those whose lives are disordered by mental illness, drug or alcohol dependence, homelessness, or migrant work patterns may have a difficult time complying with standard regimens. Those without the social support of family or friends will be challenged to continue treatment. Sometimes empathetic clinic staff can provide the needed support. Those patients who feel most in control of their own lives tend to be more compliant than those who feel they are controlled by external forces. In a treatment program for homeless persons in New York, those patients who "got back on their feet" improved their compliance with the course of treatment. Although studies of age, sex, education, socioeconomic status, occupation, or income level have shown no correlation with compliance, all groups do not have equal access to health services. People in many low paying jobs may lose a day's pay to attend daytime clinic appointments.

The degree of disability a patient suffers from an illness is directly related to compliance. The more debilitated a patient is, the more likely he or she is to comply with medical regimens.

Finally, a patient's health beliefs can have a major effect on compliance. The *health belief model* was postulated in the 1950s by Dr. Godfrey Hochbaum and his associates to explain patient compliance with medical evaluation and/or treatment (CDC, 1989). An individual's adherence to a medical regimen will be dependent on his or her perception of (a) his/her own susceptibility to the disease, (b) the seriousness of the disease, (c) the benefits of the health action, and (d) the barriers to taking the action. These beliefs have also been shown to develop during the course of an illness, as a result of the patient's early experiences during the course of treatment, thus demonstrating the importance of the patient-provider relationship from the onset of treatment.

Patients are most likely to adhere to medical regimens when the health care provider takes the time to inspire confidence through clear instructions and is able to elicit as well as give information. Frequently, denial, anxiety, and even anger will need to be addressed before a patient is ready to complete a regimen. Sometimes what the patient doesn't say can be as important as what he or she does say. More than just asking certain questions, the provider needs to read nonverbal cues and confront issues which can impede compliance and trust. Consistent follow-up with the same health care provider is the key to building such a complex relationship.

Directly Observed Therapy

An old idea recently taking on new life has been labeled directly observed therapy (DOT). When the first patients were treated with antituberculous drugs in sanitaria, every dose of medication was directly observed by the nurse administering it. Patients under treatment in tuberculosis sanitaria rapidly improved, and it was clear that hospitalization for the full course of treatment was not necessary. In the euphoria of the moment, with the scientific knowledge to cure tuberculosis readily available, it seemed that a pile of prescriptions and a few outpatient visits were all that was necessary. Tuberculosis care moved to the outpatient setting. Soon it became clear that more than a combination of the right drugs was necessary to cure tuberculosis. Multiple studies have demonstrated that patient compliance is probably the most important factor in tuberculosis cures and the most serious problem in tuberculosis control (Addington, 1979). A DOT program capitalizes on this by ensuring that a patient gets the benefit of every dose of medication. In a DOT program, the patient is initially treated in the traditional inpatient setting until he or she is stabilized on a defined regimen and is no longer contagious. During the hospitalization, the patient is observed taking his or her medications on a daily basis. After 2 to 3 weeks (assuming the organisms are sensitive to the drugs prescribed), the patient is ready for discharge. Before a patient is given prescriptions to fill and an outpatient follow-up appointment, a worker will visit the patient in the hospital to offer DOT after discharge. As discussed earlier, there are multiple reasons why a patient would not take the medicines necessary to cure his or her tuberculosis. The goal of DOT is removal of as many of these barriers as possible.

Supervised therapy, where each dose is observed, was demonstrated to be effective in a series of tuberculosis treatment failures by McDonald and colleagues (McDonald, Memon, & Reichman, 1982). Failures were defined in this study as those patients with persistently positive sputum smears for AFB for 6 months or longer after initiating therapy. All patients received supervised therapy, 5 days a week, for 6 months. In the end, 19 of 21 (90%) completed treatment. Of these patients, 14 had drug-resistant TB, and 16 were either alcohol or opiate dependent, making the success rate even more impressive.

Other studies have confirmed the efficacy of DOT used in combination with four drug regimens administered on a twice-weekly basis. In fact, this type of regimen can reduce the total number of observed doses to 62 doses in a 6-month period (Cohn, Catlin, Peterson, Judson, & Sbarbaro, 1990). The hope is that the shorter, less complicated regimens with directly observed intermittent dosing (2 or 3 times weekly) will yield higher rates of compliance and therefore higher cure rates (and fewer relapses). Fewer relapses should decrease MDR tuberculosis. A preliminary study from Texas seems to confirm this conclusion (Weis et al.,1994). Weis and colleagues found significant decreases in relapse, primary drug resistance, and secondary drug resistance after 90.5% of all tuberculosis patients were treated with DOT from 1986 to 1992 compared to self-administered regimens used from 1980 to 1986 in Tarrant County, Texas. A recent article by Frieden, Fujiwara, Washko, and Hamburg (1995) shows a 21% decrease in the number of cases of active tuberculosis in New York City from 1992 through 1994. This decline occurred primarily among those groups whose disease was thought to result from recent transmission of *M. tuberculosis*. At the same time, completion rates sharply increased because of a rapid expansion of DOT. The epidemiologic evidence suggests that DOT was responsible for the decrease in tuberculosis cases by decreasing ongoing spread of tuberculous infection. Another contributing factor for the decline may have been increased tuberculosis control efforts in institutions such as prisons, hospitals, and shelters (Frieden et al., 1995).

Studies by the Hong Kong Chest Service of the British Medical Research Council and a study in Madras, India, using entire courses of

2 or 3 weekly intermittent dosings have demonstrated successful treatment of tuberculosis in 65 to 78 doses (Hong Kong Chest Service/British Medical Research Council [HKCS/BMRC], 1987, 1991; Prabhakar, 1987). These results are equal to daily treatment regimens. Using twice- or thrice-weekly dosing from the onset greatly simplifies the task of observing medication ingestion. In addition, DOT may be more economical to administer, especially considering the fact that it can cost nearly $200,000 to treat a single case of MDR tuberculosis resulting from noncompliance or compliance with an inadequate regimen (Iseman, Cohn, & Sbarbaro, 1993).

One of the characteristics that separates DOT from other treatment programs is the use of *incentives*. Most DOT programs provide incentives to encourage compliance. An incentive can be anything that motivates a patient to complete the course of therapy. This can consist of small rewards to encourage patients to keep appointments, take medicine, or do anything else necessary to complete treatment. *Enablers* are things used to allow patients to complete therapy without which compliance would be difficult or impossible. Although the meanings of these terms sometimes overlap, in general the incentive can be thought of as more as a gift, and the enabler as a tool. Incentives can be such things as food coupons, movie tickets, a cold soda, or anything else of small value that would be valued by a patient. An enabler, on the other hand, would be something that directly enables a patient to keep an appointment, such as free transportation, or even a new car battery. These concepts are more fully explained in a pamphlet produced by the American Lung Association of South Carolina, and the South Carolina Department of Health (American Lung Association of South Carolina & Division of Tuberculosis Control, South Carolina Department of Health and Environmental Control, 1989).

Directly observed therapy is an underutilized tool to aid patient compliance and lessen the chance of relapse, drug resistance, and further spread of infection. It is now a standard recommendation of Centers for Disease Control and Prevention, The American Thoracic Society, and the American College of Chest Physicians. As its use widens, we expect to see a slowing and then a decrease in rates of tuberculous infection, disease, relapses, and drug resistance.

SUMMARY

Because of the recent increase in tuberculosis, appropriate treatment of tuberculous infection and disease has achieved a new sense of urgency. Tuberculous infection can be effectively treated, markedly reducing the rate of progression to active tuberculosis, with regimens clearly delineated by the American Thoracic Society and Centers for Disease Control (CDC, 1991a). Most importantly, this is true even for those with coincident HIV infection (Pape, Jean, Ho, Hafner, & Johnson, 1993).

The treatment of active tuberculosis has also been well described and consolidated into a brief booklet by the New York City Depart-ment of Health (1992). The main elements of tuberculosis prevention and treatment can be described in 10 basic principles, which are summarized in Table 5.4.

1. Early suspicion of tuberculosis leads to early diagnosis and treatment, helping the patient to get well sooner and protecting the community from further infection.
2. Cooperation with local health departments by reporting new cases promptly will help others treat the patient if he or she should become lost to follow-up.
3. Obtaining a careful tuberculosis treatment history can lead a practitioner to suspect and plan for drug resistance at the onset of therapy.
4. All patients should be started on all drugs, unless local rates of drug resistance are known to be very low. In New York City, as in most of the country, four antituberculous drugs are necessary for initial therapy.
5. Ongoing care needs to be consistent (follow-up visits at least monthly) and assessments of compliance are probably the most important information sought. All tuberculosis patients are candidates for HIV testing, since active tuberculosis may be a presenting sign of immunocompromise. Treatment will need to be modified for those who are HIV-infected.
6. Plan for completion of treatment at the onset. Consider DOT for all patients, especially those with demonstrated problems adhering to therapy.

TABLE 5.4 Ten Basics on the Diagnosis, Treatment, and Prevention of Tuberculosis

1. Think TB!
2. Report suspected or confirmed cases of active TB to the Health Department.
3. Always take a careful TB treatment history, and obtain drug-susceptibility studies on all initial TB isolates.
4. Begin all patients with active disease who have never been treated for TB before on at least four anti-TB drugs.
5. Ongoing care is a complex art.
6. Focus top priority on complete treatment of all patients with active TB disease.
7. Never treat MDR-TB without expert consultation.
8. Isolate hospitalized patients as soon as active TB disease is suspected or confirmed.
9. Give preventive therapy when appropriate.
10. Preventive therapy for contacts of MDR-TB cases is complicated.

Source: The New York City Department of Health (1992). Tuberculosis Treatment. *City Health Information, 11*(5), 1–4.

7. Multidrug-resistant tuberculosis needs expert consultation for management. Improper treatment can turn a curable disease into an incurable one. Tuberculosis chemotherapy should be treated as seriously as cancer chemotherapy.

8. Hospitalized patients should be isolated as soon as tuberculosis is suspected.

9. Preventive therapy should be offered to all those meeting ATS/CDC criteria for preventive therapy.

10. Preventive therapy for contacts of MDR-TB cases is complicated.

There are guidelines for treatment from ATS/CDC, which direct therapy based on factors such as

- How likely it is the patient is newly infected
- How likely it is the patient is MDR-TB infected
- How likely the patient is to develop active TB
- The drug-susceptibility pattern of the source patient's isolate

It is important to remember that drug-sensitive tuberculosis is a preventable, treatable, and usually curable disease in any patient, regardless of HIV status. HIV infection increases the likelihood of progression to active tuberculous disease, but this can still be prevented in most cases. Those with HIV disease and tuberculosis are still curable with appropriate therapy. MDR-TB carries a comparatively poor prognosis in those with HIV infection and in those with intact immunity.

REFERENCES

American Lung Association of South Carolina & Division of Tuberculosis Control, South Carolina Department of Health and Environmental Control. (1989). *Enablers and incentives.* (Available from American Lung Association of South Carolina, 1817 Gadsen Street, Columbia, SC 29201.)

Addington, W. W. (1979). Patient compliance: The most serious remaining problem in the control of tuberculosis in the United States. *Chest, 76(suppl.),* 741–743.

American Thoracic Society. (1983). Treatment of tuberculosis and other mycobacterial diseases. *American Review of Respiratory Disease, 127,* 790–796.

American Thoracic Society. (1986). Treatment of tuberculosis and tuberculous infection in adults and children. *American Review of Respiratory Disease, 134,* 355–363.

American Thoracic Society & Centers for Disease Control and Prevention. (1994). Treatment of tuberculosis and tuberculosis infection in adults and children. *American Journal of Respiratory and Critical Care Medicine, 149,* 1359–1374.

Ayvazian, L. F. (1993). History of tuberculosis. In C. Lenfant (Ed.), *Tuberculosis: A comprehensive international approach* (p. 12). New York: Marcel Dekker.

Barnes, P. F., Bloch, A. B., Davidson, P. T., & Snider, D. E., Jr. (1991). Tuberculosis in patients with human immunodeficiency virus infection. *New England Journal of Medicine, 324,* 1644–1650.

Brudney, K., & Dobkin, J. (1991). Resurgent tuberculosis in New York City: Human immunodeficiency virus, homelessness, and the decline of tuberculosis control programs. *American Review of Respiratory Disease, 144,* 745–749.

Centers for Disease Control. (1989). *Improving patient compliance in tuberculosis treatment programs.* (Available from Information Services, National Center for Prevention Services, Centers for Disease Control and Elimination, 1600 Clifton Road NE, Mailstop E-08, Atlanta, GA 30333.)

Centers for Disease Control. (1991a). *Core curriculum on tuberculosis.* Atlanta, HHS Publication #00-57630. United States Public Health Service.

Centers for Disease Control. (1991b). Purified protein derivative (PPD)-tuberculin anergy and HIV infection: Guidelines for anergy testing and management of anergic persons at risk of tuberculosis. *Morbidity and Mortality Weekly Report, 40,* 27–33.

Centers for Disease Control. (1991c). Transmission of multidrug-resistant tuberculosis from an HIV-positive client in a residential substance-abuse treatment facility. *Morbidity and Mortality Weekly Report, 40,* 129–131.

Centers for Disease Control. (1992a). Management of those exposed to multidrug-resistant tuberculosis. *Morbidity and Mortality Weekly Report, 41*(RR-11), 37–45.

Centers for Disease Control. (1992b). Transmission of multidrug-resistant tuberculosis among immunocompromised persons in a correctional system—New York,1991. *Morbidity and Mortality Weekly Report, 41,* 507–509.

Cohn, D. L., Catlin, B. J., Peterson, K. L., Judson, F. M., & Sbarbaro, J. A. (1990). A 62-dose, 6-month therapy for pulmonary and extrapulmonary tuberculosis. *Annals of Internal Medicine, 112,* 407–415.

Combs, D. L., O'Brien, R. J., & Geiter, L. J. (1990). USPHS tuberculosis short-course chemotherapy trial 21: Effectiveness, toxicity, and acceptability. *Annals of Internal Medicine, 112,* 397–406.

Daley, C. L., Small, P. M., Schecter, G. F., Schoolnik, G. K., McAdam, R. A., Jacobs, W. R., Jr., & Hopewell, P. C. (1992). An outbreak of tuberculosis with accelerated progression among persons infected with the human immunodeficiency virus. *New England Journal of Medicine, 326,* 231–235.

Dutt, A. K., & Stead, W. W. (1989). Treatment of extrapulmonary tuberculosis. *Seminars in Respiratory Infections, 4,* 225–231.

Edlin, B. R., Tokars, J. I., Grieco, M. H., Crawford, J. T., Williams, J., Sordillo, E. M., Ong, K. R., Killburn, J. O., Dooley, S. W., Castro, K. E., Jarvis, W. R., & Holmberg, S. D. (1992). An outbreak of multidrug-resistant tuberculosis among hospitalized patients with the acquired immunodeficiency program. *New England Journal of Medicine, 326,* 1514–1521.

Ferebee, S. H. (1970). Controlled chemoprophylaxis trials in tuberculosis: A general review. *Advances in Tuberculosis Research, 17,* 28–106.

Fishl, M. A., Richman, D. D., Grieco, M. H., Gottlieb, M. S., Volberding, P. A., Laskin, O. L., Leedom, J. M., Groopman, J. E., Milduan, D., & Schooley, R. T. (1987). The efficacy of azidothymidine (AZT) in the treatment of patients with AIDS and AIDS-related complex. A double-blind, placebo-controlled trial. *New England Journal of Medicine, 317,* 185–191.

Frieden, T. R., Fujiwara, P. I., Washko, R. M., & Hamburg, M. A. (1995). Tuberculosis in New York City—turning the tide. *New England Journal of Medicine, 333,* 229–233.

Frieden, T. R., Sterling, T., Pablos-Mendez, A., Kilburn, J. O., Cauthen, G. M., & Dooley, S. W. (1993). The emergence of drug-resistant tuberculosis in New York City. *New England Journal of Medicine, 328,* 521–526.

Goble, M., Iseman, M. D., Madsen, L. A., Waite, D., Ackerson, L., & Horsburgh, C. R., Jr. (1993). Treatment of 171 patients with pulmonary tuberculosis resistant to isoniazid and rifampin. *New England Journal of Medicine, 328,* 527–532.

Harris, H. W. (1994, May 6). Surgical treatment of tuberculosis. In J. Messite (Chair), *Clinical management in tuberculosis: Issues for the 1990s and beyond.* Symposium conducted at the New York Academy of Medicine, New York.

Hong Kong Chest Service/British Medical Research Council. (1987). Five-year follow up of a controlled trial of 6-month regimens of chemotherapy for pulmonary tuberculosis. *American Review of Respiratory Disease, 136,* 1339–1342.

Hong Kong Chest Service/British Medical Research Council. (1991). Controlled trial of 2, 4, and 6 months of pyrazinamide in 6-month, three-times-weekly regimens for smear-positive pulmonary tuberculosis, including an assessment of combined preparation of isoniazid, rifampin, and pyrazinamide: Results at 30 months. *American Review of Respiratory Disease, 143,* 700–706.

Iseman, M. D., & Madsen, L. A. (1989). Drug-resistant tuberculosis. *Clinics in Chest Medicine, 3*(10), 341–353.

Iseman, M. D., Cohn, D. L., & Sbarbaro, J. A. (1993). Directly observed treatment of tuberculosis: We can't afford not to try it [Sounding board]. *New England Journal of Medicine, 330,* 576–578.

Mahmoudi, A., & Iseman, M. D. (1993). Pitfalls in the care of patients with tuberculosis. *Journal of the American Medical Association, 270,* 65–68.

McDonald, R. J., Memon, A. M., & Reichman, L. B. (1982). Successful supervised ambulatory management of tuberculosis treatment failures. *Annals of Internal Medicine, 96,* 297–302.

McLaughlin, J. S., & Hankins, J.R. (1974). Current aspects of surgery for pulmonary tuberculosis. *Annals of Thoracic Surgery, 17,* 513–25.

Navarro, M. (1994, March 15). Steep drop shown in new cases of TB for New York City. *The New York Times,* p. A1.

New York City Department of Health. (1982). Tuberculosis 1882–1982: Robert

Koch and the discovery of the tuberculosis bacillus. *City Information,* 22(1), 1–4.

New York City Department of Health. (1992). Tuberculosis treatment. *City Information, 11*(5), 1–4. (Available from City Health Information, 125 Worth St., Rm 326, Box 77, New York, NY 10013.)

O'Brien, R. J. (1993). The treatment of tuberculosis. In L. B. Reichman & L. S. Hershfield (Eds.), *Tuberculosis, a comprehensive international approach* (pp. 207–240). New York: Marcel Dekker.

Pape, J. W., Jean, S. S., Ho, J. L., Hafner, A., & Johnson, W. D., Jr. (1993). Effect of isoniazid prophylaxis on the incidence of active tuberculosis and progression of HIV infection. *Lancet, 342,* 268–272.

Prabhakar, R. (1987). Fully intermittent six month regimens for pulmonary tuberculosis in South India. *Bulletin of the International Union against Tuberculosis and Lung Disease, 62*(3), 21–23.

Ryan, F. (1993). *The forgotten plague* (1st ed.). Boston: Little, Brown.

Selwyn, P. A., Hartel, D., Lewis, V. A., Schoenbaum, E. E., Vermund, S. H., Klein, R. S., Walker, A., & Friedland, G. H. (1989). A prospective study of the risk of tuberculosis among intravenous drug users with immuno-deficiency virus infection. *New England Journal of Medicine, 320,* 545–550.

Small, P. M., Schecter, G. F., Goodman, P. C., Sande, M. A., Chaisson, R. E., & Hopewell, P. C. (1991). Treatment of tuberculosis in patients with advanced human immunodeficiency virus infection. *New England Journal of Medicine, 324,* 289–294.

Snider, D. E., Layde, P. M., Hohnson, M. W., & Lyle, M. A. (1980). Treatment of tuberculosis during pregnancy. *American Review of Respiratory Disease, 122,* 65–79.

Starke, J. R. (1993). Tuberculosis in children. In L. B. Reichman & E. S. Hershfield (Eds.), *Tuberculosis, a comprehensive international approach* (pp. 329–368). New York: Marcel Dekker.

Stead, W. W., To, T., Harrison, R. W., & Abraham, J. H. (1987). Benefit-risk considerations in preventive treatment for tuberculosis in elderly persons. *Annals of Internal Medicine, 107,* 843–845.

Tuberculosis (1993, May 21). *The New York Times,* p. A1.

Vallejo, J. G., & Starke, J. R. (1992). Tuberculosis and pregnancy. *Clinics in Chest Medicine, 13,* 693–707.

Wadhawan, D., Hira, S., Mwansa, N., Tembo, G., & Perine, P. (1991). Preventive tuberculosis chemotherapy with isoniazid among persons infected with human immunodeficiency virus. In *Proceedings of the Seventh International Conference on AIDS,* Florence, Italy, June 16–21.

Walsh, J. J. (1919). The treatment of tuberculosis. In *History of medicine in New York: Three centuries of medical progress* (pp. 302–309). New York: National Americana Society.

Weis, S. E., Slocum, P. C., Blais, F. X., King, B., Nunn, M., Matney, G. B., Gomez, E., & Foresman, B. H. (1994). The effect of directly observed therapy on the rates of drug resistance and relapse in tuberculosis. *New England Journal of Medicine, 330,* 1179–1184.

6

Public Health Issues

Although no longer the threat it was in the 18th and 19th centuries, tuberculosis has been of increasing concern to the general population because of increasing numbers of cases, especially with drug-resistant organisms, in the United States and other countries as well. Throughout the world, tuberculosis is the leading cause of infectious morbidity and mortality, with increasing numbers of cases in Africa, South America and Asia. In the United States from 1953 to 1984, the annual number of reported cases of tuberculosis fell from over 80,000 to 22,255. This trend halted in 1984 and after leveling off there has been a steady increase in the annual number of new cases since 1986. As discussed earlier, this has been associated with various factors, the most important being the emergence of HIV infection. In 1989, the Centers for Disease Control (CDC) published a "Strategic Plan for the Elimination of Tuberculosis in the United States" (CDC, 1989) by the year 2010, but ever since 1985 the case rate has been rising with over 39,000 excess cases (observed versus the expected rate) by 1991. Of particular concern has been the appearance of multidrug-resistant tuberculous organisms that make treatment more difficult and may even require surgery for possible cure (Goble & Iseman, 1993). Moreover, as the disease appears more frequently, health care workers are more likely to acquire it themselves (Cornell, 1988). This has been of particular concern in New York State, with the largest numbers of cases of active tuberculosis in the United States (Adler & DiFerdinando, 1991). In 1994 Sepkowitz reviewed the subject of health care workers and their exposure to patients with tuberculosis over the last 100 years. He points out that our current view—that caring for patients with tuberculosis is an occupational hazard—emerged only in the 1950s (Sepkowitz, 1994). Many in the field felt that care of the tuberculous patient actually provided a health advantage to the health care provider. We now know that more health care workers start their employment with negative tuberculin skin tests than 100 years ago and they have no natural immunity to the infection.

RISK OF INFECTION

The greatest risk of infection arises from the subject with undiagnosed or unsuspected tuberculosis. Patients who are also infected with HIV are not more contagious than those with normal immunity but the risks to health care workers may be greater because the patients may be sicker with other HIV-related problems, which require more care, or because the patients remain contagious for longer periods.

It is difficult to give a figure for the risk of becoming infected with tuberculosis because it depends on many factors. Since it probably takes only a single tubercle bacillus inhaled deeply and implanted on the lung tissue of a susceptible host, the risk depends on the likelihood that such implantation will take place. Riley discussed this issue and pointed out that the likelihood that an airborne bacillus will be inhaled is related to the concentration in enclosed atmospheres and "hence upon the balance between the rate at which organisms are added to the air and the rate at which they are removed" (Riley, 1967, p. 623). The rate of addition depends on the type of illness (laryngeal and cavitary tuberculosis are much more contagious) and the behavior of the patient (e.g., covering the mouth when coughing), while the rate of removal depends on air circulation, disinfection of the air, and other factors. As Riley points out, "To control the rate of addition one must control the patient; control of the rate of removal involves control of the aerial environment" (1967, p. 623).

Before the availability of drug therapy, hospitals like Bellevue in New York City often had several beds filled by doctors and nurses recently infected with tuberculosis. Riley estimated that to become infected a hospital worker would have to breathe air contaminated by patients with untreated tuberculosis for 600–800 hours (Riley, 1957). Between 1930 and 1948 (pre–drug therapy) it was estimated that the average time for conversion of the tuberculin test from negative to positive in student nurses was about 1.5 years. Much quicker infection has been documented in other situations. In 1966 an outbreak of tuberculosis occurred on a Navy ship (the U.S.S. Byrd), which was well studied by Houk and associates (Houk, Baker, Sorenson, & Kent, 1968). In this outbreak, where there was continuous exposure for approximately 6 months (and not just during working hours), and where all the air was recirculated, approximately 50% of 308 enlisted personnel at risk became infected and of 66 seamen who shared a sleeping compartment with the first person with unsuspected tuberculosis, over 80% became infected.

In a more recent outbreak of tuberculosis in a housing facility for HIV-infected persons in San Francisco, Daley et al. reported that active tuberculosis developed in 11 of 30 persons, or 37% of those exposed to possible infection, and 4 others converted their tuberculin skin tests (Daley et al., 1992). Of 28 staff members with possible exposure, 6 converted their skin tests, 3 were tuberculin positive without previous skin testing, but none developed active tuberculosis. Using an analysis of the organisms recovered with restriction-fragment-length polymorphisms (RFLP), the authors could identify the first patient in the outbreak as the source of the other cases and showed that the total duration of the outbreak was only 106 days. The outbreak showed that in HIV-infected patients, recently acquired tuberculosis infections can rapidly progress to cause tuberculosis (in one patient, disease developed within 4 weeks of exposure), but also a high rate of tuberculous infection resulting from the exposure. The authors suggest that the acquisition of infection by HIV-infected residents was greater than in normal hosts.

In addition then to the number of tubercle bacilli in the air which can be inhaled is the question of the susceptibility of the host to acquiring infection with the tubercle bacillus. As noted above, it has been speculated that HIV-infected patients are more likely than hosts with normal immunity to acquire tuberculous infection when exposed to *M. tuberculosis*. We know that the explosion of tuberculosis cases among HIV-infected patients is because once they are infected with the tubercle bacillus, the infection progresses very rapidly to cause clinical disease.

Stead, Senner, Reddick, and Lofgren performed an analysis of racial differences in susceptibility to infection by *Mycobacterium tuberculosis*

(1990). They concluded, looking at infection rates among initially tuberculin-negative residents of 165 racially integrated nursing homes in Arkansas, that blacks have about twice the relative risk of whites of becoming infected with M. *tuberculosis*. This is independent of any factors which effect the progression of infection to active disease.

Obviously, avoiding exposure to airborne tubercle bacilli is the way to prevent becoming infected. What precautions should be taken while working with patients with possible or proven tuberculosis? Furthermore, should patients with tuberculosis be treated in a general hospital or a special facility? Finally, what can be done about the patient with active tuberculosis who refuses proper treatment?

Precautions

Since tuberculosis is spread by droplet nuclei which become airborne through coughing, sneezing, speaking, or even singing, precautions are directed at preventing inhalation of these infectious particles. In general these measures include (a) wearing masks, (b) sterilizing the air with ultraviolet (UV) light, and (c) ensuring proper air circulation.

Environmental surfaces are rarely a problem and special attempts to disinfect or sterilize surfaces are not necessary. This judgment would include food trays and utensils as well as objects in the room like blood pressure cuffs. A study published in 1960 showed that a hospital floor may act as a source of droplet nuclei even after a thorough cleaning (Walter & Knudsin, 1960). A short time later, Ochs suggested that dried nuclei not exposed to sunlight might be infectious for a long period of time (Ochs, 1962). This poses the problem that sweeping or cleaning a room may cause resuspension of particles. At the same time it has been shown that dried secretions are very difficult to fragment and suspend in air and that tubercle bacilli lodged on fomites do not constitute a significant infection hazard because most of them die quickly through the action of drying, and in heat and sunlight (National Tuberculosis Association Committee, 1967).

Masks

Masks can be worn by both the patient and the visitor or health care worker. Anyone with suspected or proven disease must be taught to cover their mouth and nose when coughing or sneezing, but a mask adds a further degree of protection. Since the tubercle bacillus is fairly small (2 to 10 microns), standard gauze or paper masks are not true barriers to inhaling infected particles. Particulate respirators (PRs) are used in industry to prevent the wearer from inhaling microscopic particles and various designs are in use in settings from coal mines to tuberculosis care. The National Institute for Occupational Safety and Health (NIOSH) certifies disposable PRs for industrial use and this type is now recommended by the CDC for use with patients with tuberculosis (Hutton, 1992).

The CDC has pointed out, however, that the more efficient the PR, the greater the work of breathing and perceived discomfort by the person wearing the mask (CDC, 1990). Because of this discomfort, many health care workers choose not to use PRs unless they are working in an area with cough-inducing procedures such as bronchoscopy or sputum induction. Infectious patients who leave their rooms when going for tests should wear a mask, ideally one of these more efficient PRs. The continuous wearing of masks by patients is not feasible so we must also look at other methods to clean the air of infectious particles.

Ultraviolet Lights

Ultraviolet (UV) light is part of the spectrum of electromagnetic energy generated by the sun. Air disinfection with UV light has been known since the 1930s to kill or inactivate organisms in airborne droplet nuclei, including measles, tuberculosis, and influenza bacilli. Ultraviolet lights are recommended by the CDC, but their use has been sporadic and controversial because of concern of side effects and questions about their true efficacy. We are all exposed daily to the UV in sunlight. There are actually three types of UV: A, the major type in sunlight and responsible for skin tanning, B, a minor type in sunlight which may cause skin cancer, and C, also known as shortwave UV, which includes germicidal UV (253.7 nm wavelength) used for air disinfection.

Unintentional excessive exposure of people to germicidal UV can give superficial irritation to skin and eyes with keratoconjunctivitis and skin erythema in the short term, but it is devoid of serious long-term effects (Riley & Nardell, 1989). Lights are placed as wall- or ceiling-mounted fixtures well above head level, usually 7–7.5 feet above the floor and directed to the upper air of a room, so their effectiveness depends in part upon the mixing of air in the room. Ultraviolet tubes within the fixtures should not be directly visible within 30 feet of the fixture.

Living plants are much more sensitive to light than are people and often wilt in rooms using UV light that is safe for patients and staff.

Another option is to use intense UV radiation in ventilating ducts so that recirculated air can be made germ free. This design can also be combined with high efficiency particulate air (HEPA) filters.

In addition to placement in rooms with patients with infectious tuberculosis, UV fixtures should also be used in medical settings where there is a high probability that patients with undiagnosed tuberculosis will be present. These include bronchoscopy rooms, intensive care units, and other places where procedures are done which lead to cough and airborne droplet nuclei.

Air Circulation

Various groups, including the CDC and the American Society of Heating, Refrigerating and Air Conditioning Engineers, have published guidelines for the appropriate numbers of air exchanges in various hospital areas (CDC, 1990).

In isolation rooms, air should flow from outdoors or adjacent hallways into the room with six total air changes each hour. Air from the room must then be vented outside the building away from intake vents, people and animals. Other areas, such as the intensive care units, emergency rooms, and their waiting areas, also need frequent total air exchanges. Air may be recirculated if passed through HEPA filters. As discussed above, the use of UV light in these areas adds further protection against undiagnosed tuberculosis.

In summary then, once a patient has suspected or proven active and infectious tuberculosis, he or she must be taught about the disease and the responsibility to cover mouth and nose when coughing. Staff, visitors, and the patient should use a mask when possible. The patient should be placed in a private room which is under negative pressure with the door closed. This room then draws air inward with a proper number of total air exchanges and prevents infected droplet nuclei from spreading outward to noninfected patients. Finally, UV lights should be in the room and left on 24 hours per day. The combination of these control measures will significantly reduce the chance of spread of infection.

Compliance with Therapy—Voluntary

The secret of avoiding infection is suspecting and diagnosing tuberculosis in a potential source case as early as possible. We can then protect ourselves, but it is well known that the transmission of tuberculosis can only be prevented by ensuring full compliance with therapy by patients with active disease. Brudney and Dobkin (1991) documented the extent of noncompliance in patients discharged from Harlem Hospital in New York City. They showed that in this group, 89% were lost to follow-up or failed to complete therapy. More than one quarter had to be readmitted to the hospital with active tuberculosis and most of these were again lost to follow-up.

Compliance with the full course of antituberculous therapy, as discussed in chapter 5, is the key strategy in controlling the current epidemic of tuberculosis. But in dealing with HIV infection, multidrug-resistant organisms, complex health and social problems (e.g., needs for permanent shelter, treatment for drug and alcohol abuse), how can full compliance be achieved?

Prior to the discovery of drug therapy for tuberculosis, the only therapy available was rest and fresh air. Sanatoria were available, but were mostly for terminal nursing care, until popularized by Edward Livingston Trudeau in the 1880s. The combination of rest with altitude (Trudeau's sanatorium was built in the Adirondack mountains in New York State) was later replaced with rest alone; however, patients with active and contagious disease were able to be isolated in these settings. Various forms of collapse therapy (pneumothorax, phrenic nerve crush, thoracoplasty) were also used to help put parts of the lung at rest (see Chapter 5).

With the discovery of streptomycin in the 1940s and then a multitude of drugs in the 1950s, a new form of therapy became available. Long periods of hospital care were still standard, but sanatoria were closed in the 1950s and 1960s and tuberculosis treatment moved to general hospitals. Riley, in a 1967 paper, asked whether patients with tuberculosis should be cared for in general hospitals and, if so, what precautions should be taken. The conclusion was that there was little risk to hospital personnel when proper ventilation and UV lights were used, but the emphasis was on early therapy rendering the patient non-infectious.

It is important to remember that whether a patient needs to have normal activities restricted, and the duration of those restrictions, depends on several factors. Among these are (a) the estimated degree of infectiousness (i.e., is there a small infiltrate on chest x-ray and no cough or sputum, or a large cavity with easily positive sputum for AFB?), (b) the response to treatment, (c) the nature of the activities, and (d) who will be exposed during the activity. Some patients are never infectious and therefore have no need for restrictions. Other patients who are potentially infectious can remain at home with family members who have already been exposed. It has been known for some time that once a contagious family member takes precautions against spreading tuberculosis there are usually no new cases discovered in the household. This also applies to patients who are working, especially if the environment in which they work is not conducive to transmission and there is little risk of exposure of new and/or highly susceptible contacts such as young children or patients with known immunosuppression.

Mahmoudi and Iseman reviewed common treatment errors and their association with the acquisition of drug resistance in patients admitted to the National Jewish Center for Immunology and Respiratory Medicine in Denver, Colorado (Mahmoudi & Iseman, 1993). A large part of the errors in this group of patients, many of whom were referred from other states, was due to poor physician choice of therapy. A smaller number, but still significant, were problems of noncompliance. The authors conclude that "Given the interweaving of such factors as drug resistance, immunodeficiency states, drug-drug interactions, intrainstitutional transmission, homelessness, substance abuse, and noncompliance, we submit that strong categorical programs for the treatment of tuberculosis patients may be essential . . ." (p. 68).

Compliance with Therapy—Forced

We must then look at what programs are available to ensure compliance and completion of treatment to stop the transmission of tuberculosis. Governmental power to protect the public's health and safety (known as "police power") resides in the individual states. Gostin, in early 1993, provided a 50-state survey of TB statutes and proposals for reform. He found that TB control was largely governed by "antiquated laws that predate modern concepts of constitutional law and the need for a flexible range of public health powers" (Gostin, 1993, p. 255). The major concern has been how to balance public health and human rights when dealing with an infection like tuberculosis. He reviews the duty to pay for and provide services, medical examinations, treatment (fewer than half the states specifically grant the power to impose treatment), emergency detention, commitment, isolation or quarantine, criminal penalties, and protection of patients' rights (confidentiality and antidiscrimination).

All states have the legal powers to identify infectious diseases through screening programs and require physicians and others to report the names of patients to the proper public health officials. The difficult legal problems concern the treatment of disease, especially when it includes involuntary confinement. With tuberculosis, involuntary treatment usually requires proving that someone has active tuberculosis and presents a danger of spreading it to others. Annas (1993), following reports of increasing multidrug-resistant tuberculosis, asks whether state laws should be changed to permit confinement until cure. He concludes that "the answer depends on the actual danger the patients pose to the public and the relative effectiveness of less restrictive treatment alternatives" (p. 587). The use of directly observed therapy (DOT), as discussed in the chapter on treatment, is one of these alternatives. Unfortunately the increase in cases of active tuberculosis is due to many factors, including poverty, homelessness, substance abuse, and the HIV epidemic, so that there is no easy solution to the problem of ensuring that patients complete a full course of therapy.

Nardell (1993) also has commented on the problem of conflicts between policies that favor the general good and those that favor the good of the individual when it comes to the treatment of tuberculosis. He points out that there are two groups of patients with tuberculosis in different parts of the country. First, there are those for whom the diagnosis is made quickly, treatment is effective, and the few infected contacts are promptly placed on preventive therapy. This is ideal and does not represent the problem we are seeing in large cities with high risk for multidrug-resistant tuberculosis. It is the other group that we have been concerned with in this volume, namely, those with barriers to health care who delay diagnosis and those whose treatment is inadequate. Nardell pleads that we don't lump these two groups together, but use a progressive, stepwise management approach which is appropriate to an individual patient. Starting with the least restrictive, these steps would include

1. Provide self-administered, daily short-course therapy for drug-sensitive disease with periodic follow-up in a health care facility from the very start of therapy, so that no hospitalization is necessary.
2. Provide directly observed therapy (DOT) 2 or 3 times weekly, fully supervised in the home, clinic, or alternative site. This form of monitoring would usually follow a period of hospitalization and the initial start of a more intensive regimen. It is unclear whether all patients receiving therapy for active tuberculosis should have DOT.
3. Voluntary long-term hospitalization in a specialized tuberculosis treatment unit was the normal treatment plan years ago, but it is too costly to be attractive to most public health departments. It is the last step, however, before a more enforced and formal hospitalization.
4. Finally, the most restrictive treatment plan would be compulsory, court-ordered, long-term hospitalization in a secure tuberculosis treatment unit. There is considerable literature on this subject, as discussed earlier, including the papers by Gostin and Annas.

DIAGNOSIS AND TREATMENT
IN SPECIAL POPULATIONS

The HIV-Infected Population

From the public health view, there are certain groups that pose special and unique problems in diagnosing and treating tuberculosis. At present, the largest group are those persons also infected with HIV. In this group we must suspect tuberculous infection whenever there has been exposure to tuberculosis. Use prophylactic drug therapy (usually isoniazid) whenever there is a question of infection and multidrug therapy if there is even a suggestion of active disease. Many of these issues have been discussed in earlier chapters on diagnosis and treatment. Because of the association of these two diseases, any new case of active tuberculosis should be tested for HIV. Because of the dual infection, the patients require longer periods of therapy and present even greater problems ensuring completion of therapy.

Homeless Populations

Other groups pose special problems which interfere with diagnosis and treatment. Tuberculosis in homeless populations has been extensively studied by Brickner, Scharer, and McAdam (1993). They point out that tuberculous infection and disease are relatively common among the homeless in certain cities and constituted from 10% to 27% of total cases of tuberculosis in the cities they surveyed. Based on skin testing and diagnosis of active disease, they estimated that 24% to 47% of the homeless population in various cities were infected with tubercle bacilli. A major problem for this population has been the transmission of tuberculosis in shelters, so that the longer individuals stay in the shelter system, the more likely they will be to have a positive skin test. Homelessness and unstable housing clearly lead to poor compliance with therapy. Stolen medication, long waiting times in clinics, and the prioritization of finding food and shelter above health issues impose a need for special programs to ensure compliance with therapy in this group. The most helpful strategies have been to place clinics and provide treatment in the shelters or other places where the homeless congregate. Unfortunately, an increasing number of the homeless in certain cities (e.g., New York) are intravenous drug users who also have an increased incidence of HIV infection. Thus, the potential for spread of tuberculosis in this population is quite significant.

Migrant Farm Workers

Prevention and control of tuberculosis in migrant farm workers has been addressed by the CDC (1992). They estimate that farm workers are approximately 6 times more likely to develop tuberculosis than the general population of employed adults. The category refers to seasonal workers whose transiency makes health care more difficult. Detection and diagnosis of active disease is still the number one priority. Ideally, patients should be placed on directly observed therapy given by a well-trained outreach worker from the same cultural and language background as the patient.

Institutions

Other groups that we are now targeting for special attention are residents of jails and other correctional institutions, long-term-care facilities, mental institutions, nursing homes, and other long-term residential facilities. Of these, the major problem has been in large jails and prisons, especially those with populations drawn primarily from urban areas, where increased numbers of inmates with histories of intravenous drug use and possible HIV infection have been found.

Skolnik (1992) reviewed the problem of tuberculosis in correctional facilities and pointed out that routine screening chest x-rays were now being used in various jails and prisons because of increasing reports of outbreaks of tuberculosis in prisons. He noted that there have been 11 known outbreaks from 1985 to 1992 and in one prison 13 inmates and 1 correctional officer died of multidrug-resistant tuberculosis.

Although routine tuberculin skin testing is done at most of these facilities, they are often not read or followed up properly because of a rapid turnover of inmates and many false negative results, especially in inmates infected with HIV. Furthermore an active case of tuberculosis would not be discovered for several days during which time numerous inmates and staff will have been exposed. Using screening chest x-rays on entering inmates is becoming more standard across the country. With modern equipment there is minimal radiation exposure, prompt processing, and fairly low costs. The films must be read by a radiologist on a daily basis to identify the prisoners who need to be isolated and started on therapy. At the New York City jail on Rikers Island there is now a state-of-the-art communicable disease facility to take care of inmates without having to transfer them to local hospitals.

The problem is similar but usually not of the intensity in other institutional settings, such as nursing homes and other long-term facilities.

TABLE 6.1 Goals for State Tuberculosis Control Programs

States should have systems that incorporate the following guidelines:

- Ensure the mandatory reporting of each confirmed and suspected case of TB, and observe local laws and regulations protecting patient confidentiality.

- Examine persons at high risk for TB infection and disease, prescribe the appropriate preventive or curative treatment for these persons, and monitor their treatment.

- Monitor the treatment of patients, and require that a treatment plan be devised for all hospitalized patients before they are discharged.

- Ensure the rapid laboratory examination of specimens and reporting of results to the appropriate health department and the requesting clinician.

- Ensure that TB-infected patients receive treatment until they are cured.

- Protect the health of the public by isolating and treating persons who have infectious TB and detaining persons who, although not infectious, are unwilling or unable to complete their treatment and are at risk for becoming infectious and for acquiring drug-resistant TB.

- Finance the treatment of indigent patients.

Source: Centers for Disease Control (1993). Tuberculosis control laws—United States, 1993. Recommendations of the advisory council for the elimination of tuberculosis (ACET). *MMWR* 1993;42 (No. RR-15).

populations, (b) the development and evaluation of new technologies for treatment, diagnosis, and prevention, and (c) the rapid assessment and transfer of newly developed technologies into clinical and public health practice. The role envisioned for the states is described in Table 6.1.

In order to succeed, we need to do better screening for infection, diagnose active tuberculosis as early as possible, and ensure compliance with appropriate therapy. Because of the problem of MDR tuberculosis, new drugs are needed and new tests to diagnose disease before it spreads to others must be developed. But unless state and local laws and regulations are modernized to facilitate the cure of persons with infectious tuberculosis by allowing quarantine measures including temporary confinement, this disease will continue to spread in certain areas of the country and the potential to spread more widely will increase because of the current epidemic of HIV infection.

REFERENCES

Adler, J. J., & DiFerdinando, G., Jr. (1991). Tuberculosis transmission among health care workers. *New York State Journal of Medicine, 91,* 89–90.

Annas, G. J. (1993). Control of tuberculosis—the law and the public's health. *New England Journal of Medicine, 328,* 585–588.

Brickner, P. W., Scharer, L. L., & McAdam, J. M. (1993). Tuberculosis in homeless populations. In L. B. Reichman & E. S. Hershfield (Eds.), *Tuberculosis: A comprehensive international approach* (pp. 433–454). New York: Marcel Dekker.

Brudney, K., & Dobkin, J. (1991). Resurgent tuberculosis in New York City: Human immunodeficiency virus, homelessness, and the decline of tuberculosis control programs. *American Review of Respiratory Disease, 144,* 745–749.

Centers for Disease Control. (1989). A strategic plan for the elimination of tuberculosis in the United States. *Morbidity and Mortality Weekly Report, 38*(suppl 5-3), 1–25.

Centers for Disease Control. (1990). Guidelines for preventing the transmission of tuberculosis in health care settings, with special focus on HIV-related issues. *Morbidity and Mortality Weekly Report, 39*(RR-17), 1–29.

Centers for Disease Control. (1992). Prevention and control of tuberculosis in migrant farm workers. *Morbidity and Mortality Weekly Report, 41*(RR-10), 2–12.

Centers for Disease Control. (1993). Tuberculosis Control Laws—United States, 1993. Recommendations of the Advisory Council for the Elimination of Tuberculosis (ACET). *Morbidity and Mortality Weekly Report, 42*(RR-15), 3–12.

Cornell, C. (1988). Tuberculosis in hospital employees. *American Journal of Nursing, 88,* 484–486.

Daley, C. L., Small, P. M., Schecter, G. F., Schoolnik, G. K., McAdam, R. A., Jacobs, W. R., Jr., & Hopewell, P. C. (1992). An outbreak of tuberculosis with accelerated progression among persons infected with the human immunodeficiency virus. *New England Journal of Medicine, 326,* 231–235.

Goble, M., & Iseman, M. D. (1993). Treatment of 171 patients with pulmonary tuberculosis disease resistant to isoniazid and rifampin. *New England Journal of Medicine, 328,* 527–532.

Gostin, L. O. (1993). Controlling the resurgent tuberculosis epidemic. *Journal of the American Medical Association, 269,* 255–261.

Houk, V. N., Baker, J. H., Sorenson, K., & Kent, D. C. (1968). The epidemiology of tuberculosis infection in a closed environment. *Archives of Environmental Health, 16,* 26–50.

Hutton, M. D. (1992). What is a disposable particulate respirator? *American Journal of Infection Control, 20,* 41.

Mahmoudi, A., & Iseman, M. D. (1993). Pitfalls in the care of patients with tuberculosis. *Journal of the American Medical Association, 270,* 65–68.

Nardell, E. A. (1993). Beyond four drugs: Public health policy and the treatment of the individual patient with tuberculosis. *American Review of Respiratory Disease, 148,* 2–5.

National Tuberculosis Association Committee. (1967). Statement of the National Tuberculosis Association Committee on Treatment of Tuberculosis Patients in General Hospitals. *American Review of Respiratory Disease, 96,* 836–837.

Ochs, C. W. (1962). The epidemiology of tuberculosis. *Journal of the American Medical Association, 179,* 242–247.

Riley, R. L. (1957). The J. Burns Amberson Lecture: Aerial dissemination of pulmonary tuberculosis. *American Review of Tuberculosis and Pulmonary Diseases, 76,* 931–941.

Riley, R. L. (1967). The hazard is relative. *American Review of Respiratory Disease, 96,* 623–625.

Riley, R. L., & Nardell, E. A. (1989). Clearing the air: The theory and application of ultraviolet air disinfection. *American Review of Respiratory Disease, 139,* 1286–1294.

Sepkowitz, K. (1994). Tuberculosis and the health care worker: A historical perspective. *Annals of Internal Medicine, 120,* 71–79.

Skolnik, A. (1992). Correction facility TB rates soar: Some jails bring back chest roentgenograms. *Journal of the American Medical Association, 268,* 3175–3176.

Stead, W. W., Senner, J. W., Reddick, W. T., & Lofgren, J. P. (1990). Racial differences in susceptibility to infection by *Mycobacterium tuberculosis. New England Journal of Medicine, 322,* 422–427.

Walter, C. W., & Knudsin, R. B. (1960). Floor as a reservoir of hospital infections. *Surgery, Gynecology and Obstetrics, 111,* 412–422.

Index